MAKING COMPLEMENTARY THERAPIES WORK FOR YOU

GAYE MACK, M.A.

ILLUSTRATED BY
MORGAN HESMONDHALGH

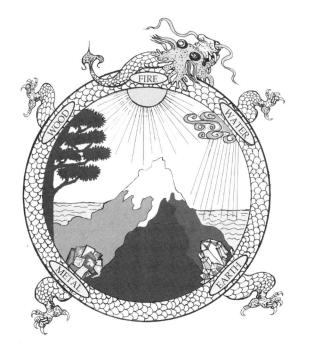

POLAIR PUBLISHING
LONDON

First Published October 2005

© Copyright, Nature's Bridge, Inc., 2005

British Library Cataloguing-in-Publication Data
A catalogue record for this book is available from the British Library

ISBN 1-905398-07-7

Author Acknowledgments
Although this is a small book, nevertheless there are those who especially deserve my appreciation for their creativity, input and clarity. First among them is Morgan Hesmondhalgh, whose very special gift for translating the author's intent into image has been proved one more time. Appreciation also goes to my long-time colleague and friend, Patricia Bright, ABT, LMT, CQGI, at the Ohio State University Center for Integrative Medicine, for her clarity on the finer points of TCM; and to James Baltzell, MD, for his insights on healing and curing. And finally,: one more physician, Jerry Gore, MD, who is responsible for getting me on this path so many years ago, deserves acknowledgment many times over.

Set in Gill Sans Light at the Publishers and
printed and bound in Great Britain by
Cambridge University Press

CONTENTS

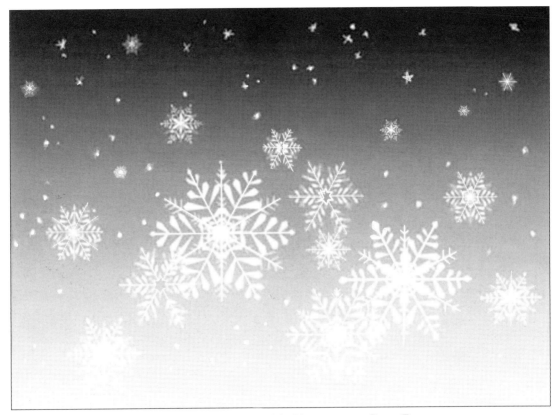

The Idea of the Microcosm and the Macrocosm—see Chapter Two

INTRODUCTION

AS MY flight from London approached Chicago, the man in the seat next to me asked if I was from Chicago. I said yes, and we began to chat. We talked about the rigours of flying. He does about 100,000 miles a year, mostly to Asia and Europe, against my paltry 40,000. I finally asked him what it was he did for a living, and he replied that he had his own company, which provides high-end optics and lasers for the medical profession.

As we chatted, he explained how he had left being a biologist to start this hi-tech company. He then asked me what I did. I laughed and told him that I was at the other end of the spectrum, as I was a practitioner and author in the field of complementary medicine. Suddenly he switched gears, and with a serious demeanour told me about the medical difficulties his wife was having.

Five years previously, when their son was born, his wife had developed a severe auto-immune disease. 'Her body is fighting itself', he said. I asked how this illness was manifesting, and he went on to say that her body was producing large amounts of histamine but that the medications to relieve the symptoms were as bad as the illness, severely altering her mood states. 'My wife is the loveliest person in the world', he said, 'but

when she takes her medication, which is needed on a daily basis, she turns into a monster'. They were desperate. They had been everywhere with no relief, and the next stop would be the world-renowned Mayo Clinic in Rochester, Minnesota, famous for its medical research and treatment of difficult cases.

As he was telling me his story, I could feel the suffering of his wife, his frustration with the irony of his background and the helplessness they felt. Stopping in midstream, he looked at me and asked, 'By any chance, do you know of someone who might help us?'. I replied that I thought perhaps I did, but made it clear that the medical practice I was going to suggest was very integrative in philosophy and application. I gave him the information as we were landing and wished them both well. He responded that they would definitely follow up on it. I hope they did.

My companion's wife is one example of the millions who, for one reason or another, have developed a chronic imbalance in their health. For some, the situation becomes so desperate that health issues dominate every aspect of their existence, severely reducing their quality of life. Along with many others, when western medicine is unable to alleviate the situation, they seriously consider therapies that do not fit this mould. In doing so, these reluctant explorers have the opportunity to reap benefit from the wisdom and value of age-old medical systems gone underground long ago.

However, this is only the beginning of the story, for the real story is in the concept of integrating old and new. This is what this book is about. It is about being careful to throw neither of the babies out with the bathwater. It is about exploring and understanding the concepts that underpin complementary therapies and how they can work for you alongside western medical technology.

HOW DO WE KNOW THEY WORK?

Western medicine places great store in 'clinical studies' or 'double blind' studies that prove or disprove the value of drugs and medical procedures. While these are extremely valuable, they can be a detriment to the acceptance of many valuable complementary therapies by western medicine. There are some therapies, such as the practice of *qigong*, which comes from Traditional Chinese Medicine, that are relatively well accepted by western medicine. Clinical studies indicate that *qigong*, for instance, 'can improve the health of people suffering from different chronic medical problems that accelerate the ageing process.... [These studies] also demon-strate that a combination therapy of *qigong* and drugs is superior to drug therapy alone [in cases of] hypertension, respiratory disease, and cancer.'*

The issue of 'clinical studies' and how relevant they are to complementary therapies is a hot one, and unfortunately too complex for this book. It should be noted, however, that western medicine, however reluctantly, but to its credit, is slowly acknowledging existing flaws in some of the most stringent of research designs; and also that there are modern drugs whose chemistry is not entirely understood to date.

In part, it is the scarcity of clinical research that is one of the basic difficulties facing the acceptance of complementary medicine by the West. Not only is there an issue of economics, but the very nature of many, if not most of these therapies is simply not conducive to the framework hard science demands. This does not mean that they are unworthy but it does mean that you must be careful in selecting the therapy and corresponding practitioner; a point that you will see repeatedly made throughout the following chapters.

It is important to understand that by calling upon the best that western medicine has to offer alongside the wisdom and practices of the ancients, we also advance in understanding our authentic selves. This, in turn, affects our perception of our environment.

* Trivieri and Anderson, ALTERNATIVE MEDICINE, p. 462.

Through this marriage, it is more than possible to experience a balanced state of health, which is essential if each of us is to manifest our life's purpose.

It is said that 'good things come in small packages'. Thus, in MAKING COMPLEMENTARY THERAPIES WORK FOR YOU, the idea is not to present you with such an abundance of information that you are more at a loss than before. The process of selecting a number of therapies to discuss in this book was difficult; complementary medicine is a huge field. In the end, I decided to look at therapies that are considered 'complete' systems of healing, as well as the compelling adjunct therapies of homeopathy and Bach Flower Remedies. The therapies chosen are also ones that are available to people living on both 'sides of the pond'. The choice of complete systems meant that some very well-known therapies, such as aromatherapy, are only scantly covered; nor could the various schools of massage be

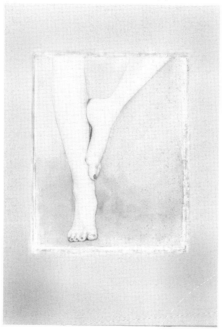

A QUEST FOR BALANCE

profiled in detail. This does not mean however, that these therapies are not valuable tools of healing. I have listed in an appendix a number of excellent books that provide in-depth information on the myriad therapies around. Such references are excellent for further expansion of understanding and study. Once one has a basic understanding of what drives the underlying philosophies of complementary therapies these references are the 'next step'.

A principle goal in writing MAKING COMPLEMENTARY THERAPIES WORK FOR YOU was to describe the underlying philosophies found in the concept of 'alternative medicine'. These basics are laid out in Chapters One and Two. Chapters Three through Six discuss the philosophies and applications of several of the major therapies; while in Chapter Seven, I have endeavoured to present a simplified explanation of what complementary therapies are talking about in reference to the 'energy of healing', yoga and meditation.

MEDITATION ALONGSIDE YOUR THERAPY

Regardless of which of the therapies or elements of the therapies discussed here appeals to you, it is important to keep in mind that mind–body–spirit philosophy is about gently getting to know your authentic self and opening up to the limitless possibilities of your highest purpose. Meditation, if you feel it is for you, is a spiritual practice and an integral element in attaining this discovery. Whether it be the more western tradition of contemplative prayer, or one of the styles of practice inherited from the East, studies show that individuals who have brought some form of spiritual practice into their lives tend to withstand better the stresses of daily life. For this reason, they are less likely to suffer from compromised immune systems that lead to illness.

It is important also to keep in mind that 'one size does not fit all' in the complementary field, which can seem vast. A therapy that works for one individual may elicit no response from another. There are several factors that go into this mix of what works and what doesn't, and in the spirit of integration, the quest for balance of mind–body–spirit is not about just one modality, but a combination.

Oh, and did I mention? In working with complementary therapies there is a hidden agenda! The one you are thinking about incorporating into your life will also take you on a journey of emotional and soul 'growth'.

GFM

Chicago, August 2005

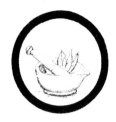

CHAPTER ONE

COMPLEMENTARY THERAPIES:

REDISCOVERING ANCIENT WISDOM

SOME TIME ago, I ran across this potted history of the evolution of medicine. Although the intent was obviously tongue-and-cheek, there is more truth in it than at first sight.

2000 B.C. Here, eat this root
1000 A.D. That root is heathen: say this prayer
1850 A.D. That prayer is superstition: take this potion
1940 A.D. That potion is snake oil: swallow this pill
1945 A.D. That pill is ineffective: take this antibiotic
2000 A.D. That antibiotic is artificial. Here, eat this root

This little book is intended for everyone who is curious about alternative medicine or new to it, but primarily the latter. It seeks to show exactly how this 'medicine' can positively impact your quality of life. Your likely images of complementary medicine, if you are unfamiliar with it, may range from the 1880s snake-oil purveyor to mysterious rituals you'd rather not think about! The reality is that these philosophies and therapies, that we also call 'holistic', are not really 'alternative' at all. Instead,

they are complementary to the medicine we have all been used to for the past several hundred years.

Complementary medicine uses some of the principles behind Granny's home remedies. Not only was Granny pretty wise, but some of her home remedies worked, and still do. In many ways, Granny was the pioneer of the revivalist movement for herbalism. Many of the herbs that she called upon are now considered mainstream, and therefore do not require discussion in the context of complementary therapy. Nonetheless, remedies like Echinacea, St John's Wort, and Arnica have been the subject of clinical research trials.

However, way before Granny's time, and even preceding the priest–physicians of the ancient world, the tribal Shaman was (and still is) the medicine man or woman, priest and negotiator in tribal cultures. While the concept of the 'Shaman' may seem strange in mainstream contexts, Shamanism is some 50,000 years old, and it is still universally revered in certain existing native cultures. This is because, inexplicably, the medicine of the tribal Shaman (which also includes elaborate rituals) has been shown to work—to the amazement of those who have studied it. Not only do the methods of Shamanism puzzle modern researchers, but the unique and ancient medical wisdoms of China and India, which we shall examine, mystify them as well. More recent therapies such as homeopathy and flower remedies can be included in a model that does not fit the western scientific framework.

The field of complementary medicine is overwhelmingly vast and constantly growing. It is a field in which previously-undiscovered therapies and their applications are still emerging. This book clarifies and systematizes information about some of the major therapies, for they have several elements in common. Essentially, they hold to a common core philosophy connecting mind, body and spirit. Furthermore, they are about lifestyle and participation on the part of the patient. Such elements are not typically part of the 'western' model, and it is to help you participate in your own wellbeing that this book has been written.

A LITTLE BIT OF HISTORY

Before we move forward, it is useful and essential to take a very brief look at the history of thought and practice which has driven holistic medicine and its therapies underground, while elevating western medicine for the past three hundred years. It is a history that begins with a kidnapping of Nature.

In the early 1600s, the world of science and medicine began to undergo a shift in the way it looked at the nature of the human condition. Scientists such as Francis Bacon, Lord Chancellor of England, began to contemplate what would happen if 'Nature' was studied from a different perspective by aggressive experimentation and observation. He and other scientific pioneers applied this method in many fields, thus revolutionizing experimental science.

Probably nowhere was the change more felt than in medicine. The new philosophy began to look at the body as a machine. In doing so, it left behind Hippocrates and the belief we associate with him, namely that body, mind, and spirit are essentially connected to health and illness. Hippocrates (460–377 B.C.E.) was a Greek philosopher and physician, and is generally considered the 'father of medicine'. He laid down rules of medicine that have lasted some two thousand years. Thus, it is no surprise that even today, physicians still 'take the Hippocratic Oath' as a rite of passage into the medical profession.

In France, the new way of thinking was taken up by René Descartes. Descartes was a philosopher, mathematician and physiologist who divined that rational thought was the only thing that was reliable. In medicine, the invariable connection between body, mind and spirit made in the tradition of Hippocrates went missing. Science embraced Bacon and Descartes, and the result has become known as the 'Cartesian split'. In a matter of a few years, their followers had pretty much lured medicine away from its traditional synthesis. Gone was the breadth of the Hippocratic vision—one, according to Dr James Gordon, author of MANIFESTO FOR A NEW MEDICINE (1996), that looked at a 'social and ecological context in which illness occurred and the way physical manifestations of disease [were] shaped by psychological and spiritual forces'.

As the wise teaching of the ancients in health matters was turned on its head, attitudes in western medicine were drastically altered and would remain so for the next three hundred years. Prior to this 'adjustment', medicine and healing had been considered an art form, first by Hippocrates' followers and then by those of Galen, who was responsible for crystallizing the best of the Hippocratic tradition in the 1500s. True physicians in this tradition focused mind, body and spirit with well-judged intent upon the healing of the mind, body and soul of the patient. With Bacon and Descartes, this inner intent on the spiritual wellbeing of both physician and patient was stripped away. Body and mind were now viewed as entirely separate entities and treated as such. Interestingly enough, our intrinsic nature compels us to search for perfect balance within, much like water seeking its own level of homeostasis. Thus, the growing interest in complementary medicine is not so surprising. Their philosophy of mind, body and spirit working in harmony, is a reflection of our innate desire to find our personal 'balance and harmony', both internally and externally.

'Complementary' is a better word than 'alternative' to describe the systems we are dealing with, for we must remind ourselves that the 'new thinking' of Bacon and Descartes (and those who followed in their footsteps over the next three hundred years) has ushered in the brilliance of what is variously referred to today as allopathic medicine, biomedicine or simply western medicine. Because it separated the body from mind and spirit, the new medicine was able to champion the idea that illness and disease should be solely treated on the basis of symptomology, rather than the more expansive view with which we are dealing in this book. While it is easy to regard the narrowing of medicine as disturbing, we must consider whether life saving discoveries in fields such as bacteriology, cardiology, immunology, neurology, obstetrics, and surgery, just to name a few, would have happened without the Cartesian split.

RECOVERING WHAT WE'VE LOST

In our own time, hardly a day goes by without the media advising us of another 'miracle breakthrough' or accomplishment in medicine. Yet for all the excitement generated, we must remind ourselves that the wisdom and methods of medicine men and women both past and present have been in danger of abandonment by the 'modern' world. Complete systems of medicine, such as traditional Chinese medicine and ayurveda, for example, are nearly five thousand years old. Even homeopathy is being developed further after two hundred years. If none of these therapies worked, would they really still be utilized by millions of people all over the world? Moreover, it is reasonable to assume that for a great many cultures outside of the West, these are the only systems of medicine called upon. If these systems did not work, surely the mortality rates would be over and above those that we are seeing as a result of famine and the diseases of poverty. Let us now see how they have come back to us.

The 1960s and 70s saw a big revolt against the whole of modernism and its ghosts. They gave us the Hippy movement, the Vietnam War protests, the Greenham Common peace camp, and they ushered in a whole new interest in the healing powers of nature that had been forced underground. Suddenly, people wanted to return to the land. They became interested in self-sufficiency and in organic farming. Thanks to teachers such as Paramahansa Yogananda and Swami Rama of the Himalayas, they rediscovered the benefits of ancient traditions, such as yoga and meditation, which had been continually practised on the Indian sub-continent. Although it was those viewed as living on the fringe of society who first took up such practices, times have changed, and these traditions and wisdoms are now more widely accepted. If we look closely, it is in these very practices that we see the principles of participation, lifestyle change, and transformation—three concepts that would, until recently, be quite unusual in allopathic medicine.

Naturally, not everyone is enthusiastic about the ancient ways, and thus not everyone will come along. Change is hard, as physicians show when they comment on positive results from a complementary therapy with remarks like, 'Well, yes, I see that it works; but if I accept that it does, I will have to change my entire way of thinking'. Only thirty years ago physicians, informed of the mental and physical benefits of yoga, laughed. Now some of them are advising their patients to go to classes. Orthodox medicine has been forced to acknowledge and to take an interest in stress-relief techniques: not only yoga but also meditation and breathing—just as much as it advises on the benefits of reducing intake of refined sugar, processed foods, dairy with hormonal additives, and replacing red meat (where possible) with a diet much closer to a vegetarian one.

For all this, western medicine has been laboriously slow in embracing alternative therapies. It tends to play a repetitive theme of the need for absolute evidence of effectiveness and safety through traditional testing techniques, while conveniently ignoring the fact that it wasn't until the 1970s that the mechanics of aspirin were fully understood. Yet aspirin, with its historical ties to the herb, willow bark, has been routinely prescribed by western medicine for decades. After recent scandals in pharmacology, once-touted miracle drugs are now suspect, tainted by adverse patient reactions and, in some cases, death.

THE ENLIGHTENED PHYSICIAN AND THE INVOLVED PATIENT

Fortunately, there are physicians in western medicine who are suggesting patients investigate holistic therapies when the tools of 'biomedicine' are not alleviating the problem. It is to their credit that they do so, as the traditional mindset of the medical schools has been that if the doctor cannot 'cure or heal' the patient, then he or she has failed. This is a heavy burden for anyone to bear, particularly a physician.

Interestingly, it is often the semantics of curing and healing that form the crossroads where western medicine and the various complementary therapies part ways. In order to understand how these therapies can work, we must start with the understanding that 'curing' and 'healing' do not mean the same thing.

In the philosophy of complementary medicine, healing is a process that can involve the healing of the inner being as well as healing of the body. Healing is an active process that requires conscious participation on the part of both practitioner and patient. This is the wisdom taught by the ancients; it is a process vastly different from the ideology of western medicine. But what does this idea of 'healing process' really mean to someone who is considering complementary therapies?

First, the process of healing requires a shift in perception and lifestyle. What was familiar practice at one time may no longer work for you. You may need to make changes to your diet, to how you manage stress, how you cope with emotional difficulties, and how you address illness when it appears. Western medicine has traditionally been practised from a directive approach. The doctor may say to the patient, 'Here, take this pill', or 'You need surgery'. Clearly, when situations call for such directives, they are wise counsel. By contrast, complementary medicine is largely preventive in nature, with a goal of your never having to face heavy medical intervention. Many of its therapies rely on nature's pharmacopoeia for support in balancing one's state of wellness, and it also incorporates therapies and practices that require your participation in body, mind, and spirit.

Equally important in the patient–physician relationship is the matter of responsibility. As you explore any therapy, it is prudent to inform your traditional healthcare practitioner of your intent. While many physicians may be uninformed about complementary therapies, there are also those who do have some degree of trustworthy knowledge about different therapies. Should your practitioner caution you, take it in consideration as wise advice with the understanding that you, the patient, are ultimately responsible for the choices you make.

According to James W. Baltzell, M.D., Assistant Professor of Radiology at the University of Minnesota, and a physician who has himself run a centre offering far more than just allopathic medicine, the greatest claims to fame that can be made for complementary therapies are in their operation on chronic illnesses. According to Baltzell, it is also the value of 'time spent' with each patient that separates the two philosophies. The economics of allopathic medicine, especially as structured along the lines of national health services, hospital and private practice corporations, and the various insurance schemes both sides of the Atlantic, do not encourage in-depth time between physician and patient. Conversely, spending quality time with each patient is an underlying core of most complementary practitioners. This philosophy deserves further discussion in the chapters that follow.

Baltzell maintains: 'Healing is related to what is going on spiritually, making your body more comfortable as you go through the difficult transits of lessons in this life. In this sense, the concept of "curing" is eradicating an acute condition that would have killed the patient a hundred years ago.… If physicians can't cure they cop out.… [In this, western] medicine is less effective in the long run.'

Nevertheless, it is foolish to declare that either approach is better than the other; each deserves respect in its own place. There are situations when 'trauma medicine' is required. If you are in crisis from a heart attack, you need the brilliance that western medical technology has produced. However, there are also complementary therapies that can assist you in the process of your recovery, after the crisis has passed. Utilizing the best of both of these worlds brings us to the concept of integration. When, in medical crisis, we embrace the best that both complementary and allopathic medicine have to offer, then we in turn are being holistic: doing the very best for ourselves on the road to healing.

WHERE TO SEEK HELP

Complementary medicine is not just about where to turn in the event of a breakdown in your health.

The philosophy upon which complementary medicine relies offers a deeper and broader approach to our wellbeing than that. In matters of health and healing, its belief that we are spirit in body offers a series of layers through which disease can manifest. What affects us negatively, both emotionally and spiritually, will eventually manifest physically.

From a practical standpoint, there are several distinctions in methodology and core philosophy between allopathic and holistic medicine. Depending on the country, professionals who practise in the various specialties of allopathic medicine are identified by recognizable letters following their names. These identifiers not only indicate years of advanced study, but may also imply the granting of a licence to practice by governing bodies. While there are those with a traditional medical background who have incorporated complementary therapies into their practice, the majority of practitioners in complementary medicine may not carry such credentials, simply because in some parts of the world, the framework does not exist for such licencing.

It is important, therefore, to clarify that lack of familiar credentials such as M.D. does not mean that a complementary practitioner has not had years of education, practice, and expertise. For holistic practitioners, credentials are typically awarded by institutions whose focus and education is in one particular modality or specialty. In America, the issue of licensing has become a heated source of debate for many highly-qualified complementary practitioners who have years of knowledge and experience behind them. Sadly, they are often unable to practice within an institutional setting such as a hospital for lack of a licence; a frustrating situation.

Thus, when you are in search of a practitioner of alternative medicine, it is wise to make some sort of investigation of the practitioner along with the therapy. The first matter of importance is to clarify the soundness of his or her credentials, whatever they may be. Considerations could include the reputation of the certifying body. What are the requirements for any certification or professional designation? Referral by people whom you trust is one of the best sources of investigation before you walk through the door of any therapist's office. Furthermore, read up on the therapy you are interested in. As you may discover in the pages that follow, choosing a holistic therapy that is a right fit for you is not unlike getting engaged; time is going to help develop an integrative relationship between the therapy, the practitioner and most importantly, you, the patient.

This is a key difference between it and the relationship you have with allopathic medicine, even though you may prefer one doctor's suggestions before another's. Additionally, you may discover that as you move forward in your healing process, the complementary therapies you once chose or the specific elements within them, may no longer apply, requiring a change. This is perfectly normal; in some instances it may be an indication that you are moving forward. Furthermore, when you choose to incorporate complementary therapies into your personal healing model, it is common to work with elements found in more than one therapy, for healing is an alchemical process. It is a process that compels you to connect to your internal landscape, not simply as an overview, but it becomes an excavation of your 'authentic self'. Moreover, it is in this excavation that we discover our highest good and purpose.

All in all, MAKING COMPLEMENTARY THERAPIES WORK FOR YOU is a matter of participation, awareness, reflection, and growth. That is to say, participation in any of the therapies tends to require that you have made the decision to take a hands-on role in your healing. Inclusive systems such as traditional Chinese medicine, ayurveda, or homeopathy are not to be compared with the so-called 'magic bullet' syndrome. Embracing these systems of healing requires that you take a committed interest in your process. Traditional Chinese medicine and ayurveda, for example, often fashion an individual plan for you known as a 'protocol'. Your protocol might include various herbal teas, perhaps some remedies, stress-reduction techniques, and dietary changes. Each of these is necessary as they interact in important ways. The good news is that you will find, by understanding and participating in what is expected of you, that the discoveries of reflection, awareness, and growth, will naturally come as part of the healing process.

KEY POINTS OF CHAPTER ONE

- Complementary or holistic medicine and its therapies is about integration of our mind–body–spirit.
- Many complementary therapies have foundations in ancient systems of healing.
- Complementary medicine and allopathic medicine can and do work in an integrative manner.
- Complementary medicine requires participation by both practitioner and patient (client).

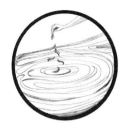

CHAPTER TWO

DON'T SHOOT THE MESSENGER:

THE MESSAGES WE GET FROM ILLNESS

IN THE ANCIENT world, if you had a career as a messenger, you were in a tricky business. If you delivered good news to upper management, you had short-term job security until the next assignment. Conversely, if you arrived with bad news, your prospects for further employment were precarious, at best. The bottom line is that your fate rested on the interpretative perspective of your message by upper management.

Complementary medicine is much more likely than biomedicine to see illness as a message. Presently, the hi-tech environment in which much of the world functions is filled with messages. Our lives are ordered by text messages, email messages, phone voice-mail, post-it notes and written memos. But despite the messages we expect, there are messages that we often never hear at all. These are the messages that are presented to us by our higher wisdom, some of which are cloaked in the guise of illness. When confronted with chronic health situations affecting our quality of life, we tend to place all of our focus on the symptoms, oblivious to the larger picture.

In mind–body–spirit philosophy, we don't always get what we want: we get what we need. This is a key tenet in holistic medicine. In other words, the philosophy and the medicine go hand in hand, and they are interacting consistently when we pay attention to the signals illness brings. Sometimes their purpose is to raise our awareness to mis-steps we are taking within our lives. Such steps block us from manifesting our highest purpose. As I pointed out in the previous chapter, any disharmony that exists in our external lives may be mirrored in our emotional and physical selves. Examining this helps us understand the connection between mind, body and spirit, and states of harmony and disharmony.

Now, you may be thinking, 'Uh, oh. I need to make changes'. Yes, this is true. But, before you plummet into depression at the very thought, know that this is really good news—in fact, great news. Each block we create in our internal and external world has a red flag on it the moment illness manifests, alerting us to the fact that we need to make changes in order to move forward. As human beings we like to stay snug in our comfort zone, and without such prompts, 'change' is not something we readily embrace.

This is good news, but it is not new news, of course. While the Cartesian split has sidetracked the concept for the past thee hundred years, the mind-body-spirit philosophy of Hippocrates' day is now enjoying a well-deserved second showing, under various names. In the scientific community, the philosophy is typically referred to as PNI or psychoneuroimmunology. In the popular field, you will more often hear 'complementary medicine', 'alternative therapies', 'holistic medicine', 'mind-body-spirit medicine', or 'natural therapies'.

If, for a moment, we consider complementary medicine as a 'holistic' model for healing mind–body–spirit, then we are in sync with the Hippocratic philosophy of treating the whole person. This means the inclusion of healing mind and spirit, rather than just addressing physical illnesses. It may help to keep in mind that in orthodox western medicine, 'matter' is primary; but in the traditions from which many of the alternative therapies originate, 'consciousness' is primary. In other words, in complementary medicine, reconnection to our spiritual self is what healing body and mind is about. When we adopt this model, we become engaged in a continual process that has a goal of total balance between body, mind, and spirit. It is in this process that we have many therapeutic tools to choose from on our journey. Many of these tools have aspects that can work on one, two, or all three levels, as illustrated below:

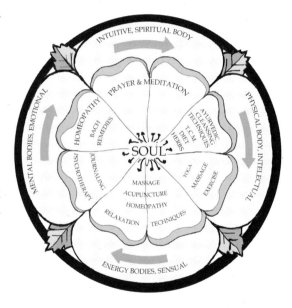

THE ALCHEMY OF BALANCE BETWEEN MIND, BODY AND SPIRIT

AN UNDERLYING ORDER

Some of the traditional systems that have made a transition to the West, especially those rooted in the Far East and India, incorporate the concept of five spiritual laws into daily life. While it is not imperative to embrace the concepts of these laws in order to benefit from the wisdom of complementary therapies, it is useful to consider them for brief discussion in order to understand how they work in our lives and how they may be interpreted through the messages that illness has for us. They are a sort of 'common stock' from which many assumptions tend to be made in the holistic field, directly or indirectly. To some extent they come from the Vedic wisdom (see Chapter Three), which is some of the earliest wisdom we have, and take their present form through Hinduism.

A quick look at them may explain more about complementary therapies than in-depth study of the therapies themselves can.* The laws introduce us to the concepts of *Karma*, Rebirth, Opportunity, Correspondence, and Balance. In one way or another, each of the major systems of medicine covered in the following pages incorporates one or more of these laws. Some philosophies place a great importance on them while others only give them a vague reference. The purpose of mentioning them here is that should you come across references to them in your researches, the language will not have you shoving the book back on the shelf or abandoning the therapy! So, here we go.

The first of these laws are those of Rebirth and *Karma*. It affirms that as spirit in a body, we incarnate through a cycle of many physical lives. The belief is that this cycle of rebirth is necessary in order that we learn earthly lessons essential to soul growth and eventual illumination. Illumination is the Golden Apple of the spiritual seeker, and it comes from unconditional surrender to the wisdom of the Divine in every cell of our physical bodies and the external world, and in every vibration of our etheric bodies.* It is the ultimate connection we make with all that is Divine within and without us. Thus 'enlightened', we come to recognize our high truth, our soul purpose.

However, there is a catch to the law of Rebirth and that is *Karma*, also referred to as the law of 'Cause and Effect'. Within each incarnation, we are responsible for our thoughts and actions, both positive and negative. We are accountable for both kindnesses we have extended (deposits in our karmic 'bank account') as

*These laws are not specifically eastern. For a recent perspective, see WHITE EAGLE ON LIVING IN HARMONY WITH THE SPIRIT (White Eagle Publishing Trust, Liss, Hampshire, 2005).

*Chapter 7 explores the concepts of 'etheric' and 'energy channels'.

well as unkind thoughts or acts (debits). This is notable in holistic systems: the idea that thoughts are powerful for good or ill as well as deeds. Our 'bank balance' rolls over to each incarnation so that in the end all debits require payment in full through transformation into acts of love and kindness.

Of the five laws, *Karma* is probably the one that people are most familiar with, but their understanding of it is not always accurate. For instance, those who have incarnated into this life with birth defects or disabilities may well wonder why this has happened to them. Similar questions come when people are faced with a life-threatening illness they seem not to deserve. They ask themselves, 'What did I do to deserve this *karma*?' Yet from the perspective of spiritual law, the issue is not punishment, but growth and opportunity. A couple of examples will demonstrate what great opportunities sometimes exist in these restrictive situations.

At the age of 42 and at the height of his career, the actor, Christopher Reeves, was irreversibly paralyzed by an equestrian accident witnessed by a horrified audience. Reeves fought to recover from his condition with determination, but it was not to be, as he recently died. Secondly, in August 2005, Peter Jennings of ABC World News, known globally to thousands for his brilliant reporting, died after a brief fight with lung cancer.

From the short view, we look at the loss of these two men as senseless and undeserving. From the longer perspective, it is quite another story. Because of his high profile as an actor, Reeves was able to bring much-needed attention to the plight of quadriplegics, particularly in the field of spinal injury research. After Peter Jennings' death, ABC Television was immediately flooded with thousands of emails from viewers, vowing to give up smoking. The American Cancer Society reported a similar volume of response, to the extent of saying that even if a small fraction followed their determination, as many as five hundred lives a week would be saved. These two men couldn't possibly know the extensive effects that their personal situations would have upon the lives of others, whom they would never meet.

Karma is thus bound up with the next law, that of Opportunity. It ensures us that during each incarnation, we have the opportunity to 'work' our karmic bank account. The opportunities come within the framework of life-experiences and through those who come into our lives. Sometimes an individual who has been suffering from a chronic condition will be quick to blame his or her illness on circumstances or individuals with whom the individual must interact. The law of Opportunity is there to teach us that the things we find challenging are actually a creation of our soul's wisdom so that we may grow by overcoming them through time.

If you find these three laws difficult to embrace, do

not worry too much, because it is the laws of Correspondence and Balance that are the most aligned to holistic ideas about the context of illness, and the philosophy behind alternative medicine and its therapies. We met one aspect of the law of Correspondence in the previous chapter, when I described the need for balance between the macrocosm (our external environment) and the microcosm (our internal environment). It is also reflected in the way minute components of our bodies contain the blueprints of the whole. To re-emphasize, the philosophy of holistic medicine infers that if our body is out of balance, we only have to look to our relationship to our external environment as to 'probable cause'. The clues will be there, giving us opportunity to make different choices in behaviour patterns.

In the law of Balance, we meet this larger picture: the issue of humanity being in balance with the cosmos. All of nature works within this law, through such polarities as positive/negative, dark/light, and silence/sound. According to Joan Hodgson, author of ASTROLOGY, THE SACRED SCIENCE, this Law 'ensures that all life develops according to its own rhythms. The whole Cosmos is held in a state of perfect balance by the polarity of opposites'. Thus, by working with both allopathic medicine and its alternatives (themselves seeming opposites), we are working for balance within us on the levels of mind, body, and spirit.

Thus, regardless of your personal beliefs, these concepts can be applied in the broadest sense of the dynamics that are the foundation of complementary medicine. Like all of nature, we are a form of energy, and when we become ill, it is because there is a blockage in the normal flow of energy within our bodies. Thus, in order to heal, these blockages need to be removed. In doing so, holistic practitioners will call upon various approaches such as acupuncture, massage and/or exercise such as yoga, tai chi, and *qigong*. These methods work to balance the channels of energy that surround and are within the body. Others will utilize different forms of remedies that fall under the category of 'vibrational medicine' such as homeopathy and flower remedies. Additionally, there are other alternative areas in which practitioners work, including Herbal Medicine, Aromatherapy, and various forms of meditation.

While the general field of complementary therapies is vast, the chapters that follow will explore the specific characteristics of several major modalities and philosophies. It is important to note that no matter which of the therapies you chose, whether from those explored here, or those you explore on your own, there is no body of reference that should be considered a replacement for working with a qualified practitioner. It must be remembered that much of allopathic medicine has its roots in the older traditions. Just because a therapy is ancient does not mean that working with it does not require guidance and supervision by a qualified practitioner with years of education and experience.

Having heard this caution, we now can begin with the two ancient cousins of eastern medicine: the traditions of Chinese medicine on the one hand, and Ayurveda, which comes from India, on the other.

CHAPTER TWO KEY CONCEPTS:

• Illness can be a message to us that gives us an opportunity to make changes in our perceptions and lifestyles.
• Alternative medicine is a 'holistic' model for healing and achieving balance on the levels of body, mind, and spirit.
• Connecting to our spiritual self is just as important as healing our body and emotions.

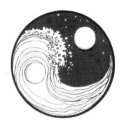

CHAPTER THREE

TRADITIONAL CHINESE MEDICINE:

A FOUR-PILLAR MODEL

TRADITIONAL Chinese Medicine (TCM for short) originated in an agrarian culture at least 3,500 years ago. From a western perspective, the philosophy of traditional Chinese medicine is 'alternative' in how it addresses illness and in the therapies used to treat illness. TCM recognizes that humanity is an element of nature. Much of its framework is said to be derived from Taoist philosophy, which covers many areas including freedom, nature, cosmology, and personal growth. Like those in the natural world, the elements within us as humans ebb and flow internally as well as externally.

Although scholarship holds the origins of TCM to be more recent, Chinese tradition teaches that it was originally formulated by Huangdi, the Yellow Emperor. Traditionally, Huangdi lived from 2698 to 2598 B.C.E. and wrote a treatise entitled *Neijing Suwen*, which means 'Basic Questions of Internal Medicine'. Near the end of the second century C.E., an official named Chang Chung-Ching wrote his 'Treatise on Typhoid

Fever', containing the earliest known reference to *Neijing Suwen*. Furthermore, historians inform us that Wang Ping (Tang dynasty, 618-907 C.E.) substantially edited and expanded the *Neijing Suwen* from copies he claimed to have located. The result is believed to be the foundation of TCM.

According to ALTERNATIVE MEDICINE, THE DEFINITIVE GUIDE (Trivieri and Anderson, 2002), a quarter of the world's population uses one or more of TCM's therapies, which seems astonishing. It would be safe to estimate that since that statement was made, the number of its advocates in the West has grown, as still more of us embrace aspects of this very old medical tradition.

TCM is sometimes offered as oriental medicine. Technically, 'oriental medicine' includes methods and techniques from other areas of Asia and India. Rather than a single therapy, it is a complete system that looks at the body as a whole system in terms of how it is, or is not, functioning. As an analogy, we can think of an illness represented by a tree with its branches and roots. TCM treats the branches (symptoms), as does western medicine, but most importantly it looks to discover and treat the primary or underlying cause (the root) of the imbalance. The complete system of TCM can seem overwhelming to the uninitiated, so it is useful to look at some of the basics involved in the tradition.

TCM identifies major 'pillars' in its model of healing. These include herbs, massage, acupuncture and *qigong*. As it is a vast system, we need to keep in mind that even within these major therapies or modalities there are some variations—depending on how and where the physician has received his or her training. As a result, practitioners of TCM carry a variety of credentials. For example, an OMD (Oriental Medicine Doctor) has had to complete years of complex education and examination, similar to the MD designation in western medicine. In addition, there are practitioners who have been certificated (and depending on location, licensed), to practise one or more therapies within the field, such as acupuncture and various massage therapies.

How you choose a practitioner who is well qualified is important, as with any complementary therapy (see Chapter One). A combination of research into his or her educational background and qualifications as well as personal recommendations, is an excellent approach. Choice of physician or therapist is just as important as

the therapy, because during your healing process, you will forge a partnership with your practitioner as he or she also teaches you preventive self-care.

If the large umbrella of TCM seems daunting at first, it is quite possible to gain benefit by incorporating just one or more of TCM's therapies into your lifestyle. You can gain much benefit by doing this fairly simply, even slowly, choosing one at a time. However, before discussing the main therapies within TCM, we should first have a brief look at the overall philosophy.

TCM is not simply a system that offers curative approaches to illness but also a preventive system, working from the belief that if balance in mind, body, and spirit can be maintained, illness and disease will not develop. TCM functions in harmony with the holistic philosophy that the state of our body is a reflection of how well we are connecting to our external environment. In TCM, our body is part of the natural world, and as such it is a reflection of our personal world as well. Either we flow along energetically in harmony or, for various reasons, we become blocked and stagnant within. When this happens, we have set up an inviting environment for illness to take hold; not a good thing.

As you begin to investigate whether or not TCM is for you, you will initially come across several terms that are native to TCM. Among the first is *qi* (sometimes spelt *chi*). *Qi* refers to the 'vitality', or 'life-force' that enlivens the universe and all things within the universe. *Qi* flows within the body through an invisible network of channels called meridians. 'Meridian', as used in TCM, may seem an unusual word to use: it is a translation from the Chinese term, *jingluo,* into French, then English. '*Jing*' means 'to go through', *luo* means 'something that connects or attaches. Separate from blood vessels, meridians are pathways or channels just below the surface of the skin. There are fourteen main meridians flowing throughout the body and their function is to connect what the Chinese identify as the 'fundamental substances'.* These substances include *qi*, blood, fluids, *jing* and *shen.* We cannot look at these in great depth,† but suffice it to say that while the balance of each fundamental substance is necessary in TCM, it is the 'vital life-force', the *qi*, flowing through the meridians that support our emotions, mental attitudes and organs with nourishment and strength. It is the subtle strength or weakness (blockage)

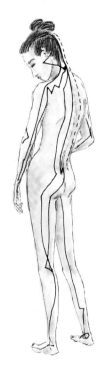

along the meridian pathway that leads to disharmony within us.

When *qi* is very weak, we may have difficulty with digestion or energetic output. When *qi* is excessive, we may find that we react with anger or fear in an excessive manner. Over time, imbalances in the *qi* flow create a disintegrative effect, which may create an open doorway for illness to step through. Finally, it is important to underscore that the meridians can become blocked for a variety of reasons. External causes could include pathogens or germs, while internal causes can stem from emotional distress.

YANG, YIN AND THE FIVE ELEMENTS

Two other words native to TCM are *yang* and *yin.* According to Ted J. Kaptchuk, OMD, author of THE WEB THAT HAS NO WEAVER, *yang* and *yin* are not forces such as energy, nor are they material, but in fact are 'convenient labels to describe how things function in relation to each other and the universe'. *Yang* is generally considered active, light, and hot, while *yin* is receptive, dark, and cold. Additionally, *yang* often refers to the

*Kaptchuk, Ted J., THE WEB THAT HAS NO WEAVER, pp. 77, 34–46.
†See 'Suggested Reading' for recommendations as to how to explore this subject in depth.

universal male principle and *yin* to the feminine. Each is essential for the other to exist. For example, we cannot know what 'light' is if there is no 'dark' to compare it with; nor what heat is, if we have not experienced cold. Thus all of nature, including ourselves, functions in this chronic balancing act. The question is, how well are we really functioning?

Qi, being the element of connection between all things, is either *yang* or *yin*. Thus, *yang qi* is masculine in nature, dynamic, and fiery; the energy that moves and motivates. *Yin qi* is receptive, passive and calming, like a still pond or lake. In TCM, a patient's *yin–yang* balance is evaluated accordingly. Thus, the physician or practitioner assesses the patient on many levels, taking in various aspects of his or her environment, lifestyle, history, and emotional outlook, which is why TCM is an extremely individualized tradition.

TCM is also grounded in everyday life and the environment in which we live; every part of the whole has a synchronistic connection. There is another aspect of TCM that assigns an elemental nature to how our organs function in relationship to one another in supportive and controlling roles, as shown in the illustration.

In looking at the arrows around the outside of the petals in the diagram, we can see how each organ with its assigned element supports another. For example, kidney (water) supports the liver (wood). Liver (wood)

supports the heart (fire), and so on. But each organ also regulates the balance and imbalances of *qi* in another organ, as indicated by the internal arrows. Thus, the lungs (metal) regulate the *qi* in the liver (wood), the liver (wood) regulates *qi* in the spleen (earth), and the spleen (earth) regulates the *qi* of the kidneys (water) that in turn regulates the *qi* of the heart (fire). Each organ passes energy to another and it also responsible for regulating any imbalances of *qi* in another.

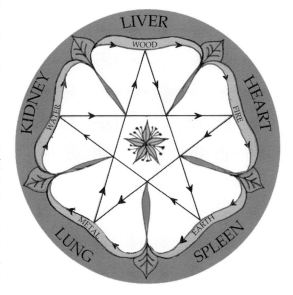

Never forget that TCM offers a complete system of medicine embodying centuries of medical wisdom. Furthermore, the starting-point of this system is how we connect to our external and internal worlds, and how they in turn, relate to each other. To a practitioner of TCM, if we are out of balance with our intended nature in mind, body and spirit, then we are in a state of disharmony with the flow of nature around us.

THE FOUR PILLARS

This now brings us to a brief exploration of the major therapies used for treatment in TCM. Essentially, they are herbal medicine, acupuncture, massage, and *qigong*. Diet is not discussed in detail in this book, but it should be understood that a balanced and nutritious diet is an essential element of support, regardless of what particular therapy or therapies are called upon. It is impossible for the body to heal if we ignore diet and nutrition.

Herbal medicine is used in every major culture around the world, and has been for thousands of years. In many cases, the wisdom of uses and secret formulas have been passed down from generation to generation, including the wisdom and methods of Granny's home remedies, mentioned in Chapter One.

Herbs are central to the practice of TCM, with the knowledge having been preserved in pharmacopeias dating back to the early Han dynasty (third century B.C.E.). However, a TCM physician may use a formula of up to nineteen ingredients, selected to treat both the branches and root of our tree, the metaphor previously used. These ingredients can come from a variety of sources in the plant, mineral, and animal kingdoms. Some ingredients will be familiar to us, others seemingly quite peculiar. The individual ingredients within the formula must be in balance with each other, or else the formula will not be as effective as intended or perhaps even counterproductive.

Herbal concoctions are typically administered in the form of teas, that can taste like something you'd rather not discuss in mixed company. However, they are also administered in the form of pills, powders, tinctures, and poultices, which, depending on the herbal concoction, can be a saving grace. According to Dr. Maoshing Ni, President of Yo San University of Traditional Chinese medicine, Marina Del Rey, California, 'What defines mastery in Traditional Chinese Medicine, is the ability of the practitioner to formulate complex combinations of various herbs for a collective purpose. The herbal formulation is often different for every patient due to TCM's personalized objective. That is the beauty of Traditional Chinese Medicine—to tailor the treatment to each individual patient's needs.'

Acupuncture is another therapy extensively used

in TCM, and involves the placement of very fine needles into specific points along the meridians. Although acupuncture recognizes thousands of these points, a practitioner's repertoire is typically made up of not more than a hundred and fifty, if that many, and a single acupuncture session usually involves as few of them as the treatment will permit.

The theory behind acupuncture is that each point has an action of its own, one that is essentially therapeutic. Acupuncture is considered a *yang* therapy, one of action, as it moves from the exterior to the interior. The practitioner determines which points to work on according to the specific disharmony of the patient. Inserting the needles only a millimetre or two into the point rebalances the flow of energy within the meridian, thus relieving pain or facilitating restoration of health to the patient.

While the very thought of having needles of any sort embedded in you may be enough to spoil your appetite, material used to make acupuncture needles has evolved, over the centuries. Originally it is thought that they might have been made of materials such as bone, horn, or bamboo, and later of bronze and other available metals. Acupuncture needles of today are made of stainless steel, thin as a strand of hair and hardly felt: definitely an improvement!

When the practice of acupuncture first appeared in the West it was, like many complementary therapies, dismissed by the biomedicine community. Recently, though, numerous scientific studies have shown its effectiveness in bringing relief to individuals who have suffered from chronic pain or illness but have not responded to western medicine. Thus, the West is now finding it essential to recognize acupuncture as a viable and extremely valuable therapy.

If, despite the improvement in the materials used for its needles, acupuncture is still too much for you to consider, the massage therapies used in TCM may instead sound appealing. In TCM, there are a great many disciplines of massage therapy, including osteopathic and chiropractic approaches. In addition to these more 'vigorous' methods, there are others that use finger pressure to promote the flow of *qi*, in order to remove blockages. Unlike western styles of massage, which use techniques of kneading and friction, these methods work by applying finger pressure on the acupuncture points along the meridians and gently stretching the limbs.

Typically, since western methods of massage utilize various types of massage oils, the individual is asked to remove all or most of their clothing for the treatment. By its nature the finger-pressure massage used in TCM does not require removal of clothes for a completely effective treatment. The massage used in TCM can thus be very appealing to those uncomfortable with the western approach, as it is non-invasive.

The last of the pillars of TCM is *qigong* (chi kung), which is a form of energy healing. Those unfamiliar with the concept of the body's energetic fields should refer to Chapter Seven—since it is at the core of several alternative therapies. While in TCM there are several traditions of energy healing used by practitioners, generally they all focus on working with the body's energetic fields. *Qigong* involves learning body movement patterns that are usually taught by a qualified practitioner or Master. Thus, *qigong* engages and requires your full participation, as it evolves into your personal 'practice'.

Qigong is time-honoured in TCM and thought to be at least 4,000 years old. In this tradition, we are working with our *qi* as both a participant and/or patient in an effort to bring balance, harmony, and health into our daily life. Medical *qigong* involves both internal and external techniques that include meditating, cleansing, strengthening and recharging, circulating, and dispersing *qi*. You can also learn to practice *qigong* as a means to spiritual growth or self-awareness, and it can be practised as a martial art.

Another energy therapy traditional to TCM is tai chi (*taijiquan*), sometimes described as a moving form of yoga and meditation combined. Many of the movements or 'forms' of tai chi come from the martial arts, but in tai chi, movement is intentionally slow and graceful, including the transitions between forms. The goal of tai chi is for the individual to cultivate a calm and tranquil state of being while focusing on precise execution of the forms. In addition, the forms themselves can also promote strengthening of muscles and skeletal posture.

Meditation, in the context of both *qigong* and tai chi, may not appeal to you at all. Do not despair, for as I mentioned previously there are many approaches to meditation. These are but two of many paths to the practice. The world is full of traditions and practices that incorporate 'meditation', ranging from developed forms of prayer in the western religions, through 'mindfulness meditation' as practised in some forms of Buddhism, to the way meditation is taught in the extensive system of yoga. As we explore the specifics of some of these approaches in the chapters that follow, you will see there are many alternatives available to you. However, regardless of which approach of meditation you find comfortable to work with, the basic role of meditative practice, as it relates to complementary medicine, is to assist you in stress-reduction, relaxation, and reconnection with your highest purpose.

Clearly, traditional Chinese medicine has a lot to offer in its wisdom and in its various therapies. However, it cannot be restated strongly enough that care in choosing a physician or practitioner is paramount. Secondly, as with most alternative therapies, in order to gain full benefit from any of your healing process, you must be a participant, not an observer. When you participate fully, the benefits you can gain are priceless.

We now move from the Far East to India, home of ayurvedic medicine.

CHAPTER THREE KEY POINTS:

- TCM is at least 3,500 years old.
- The uninterrupted flow of *qi* through the meridians is essential to our state of wellness in body, mind, and spirit.
- Using the five elements of water, fire, earth, air, and metal our ten major organs support each other in the flow and balance of *qi*.
- Herbs, acupuncture, massage, and *qigong*, as both a form of movement (exercise) and hands-on healing, make up the four pillars of TCM.
- Considerable care is essential in choosing a physician or practitioner of TCM.

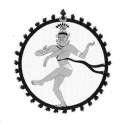

CHAPTER FOUR

AYURVEDIC MEDICINE:

WHAT YOUR *DOSHA* IS TELLING YOU

EAST MEETS West in the healing philosophies of Chinese medicine, in eastern Asia, and those of *Ayurveda*, native to India, Tibet, and other countries in southern Asia. Logically, it might seem that these two systems of medicine would differ from each other, given the diversity among the cultures that practise them. The reality is that at their roots they are more alike than not.

Ayurveda 'is a comprehensive system of medicine that combines natural therapies with a highly personalized approach to maintaining health and the treatment of disease. [It] places equal emphasis on body, mind, and spirit, and strives to restore the innate harmony of the individual'.* Ayurveda's philosophy, like TCM's, focuses on the subtle energy that exists in all forms of nature, both organic and inorganic. Its practice extends further to our thoughts and emotions, through the inclusion of yoga and meditation, both of which have an effect on our state of wellness.

*Trivieri and Anderson, p. 86.

Here we have another example of a comprehensive system of medicine and healing requiring patient participation. However, to gain a basic understanding of how ayurvedic medicine views illness and healing, we need to look at the whole Indian tradition, its origin.

A large portion of India's culture is grounded in ancient Hindu scriptures known as *Vedas*. According to Rudolph Ballentine, M.D., author of RADICAL HEALING, spiritual practice as laid out in the original Vedas did not include emotions or the body. Later adaptations however, evolved into what is known as tantric philosophy. More advanced in its perception of the universe, this philosophy professed a greater reverence for the feminine principle and was very much in tune with the concept of subtle energy.*

Additionally, the later versions of tantric philosophy incorporated the five elements. We find similarities again to traditional Chinese medicine, except that

*Ballentine, RADICAL HEALING, p. 586.

tantric philosophy includes the element of ether rather than the element, metal. In Hindu mythology, the god Shiva explains to his lover, Parvati, that all we 'see and know emerged from a blending of the Five Elements or *tattvas*. They are the subtle bases of all that is physical and energetic … or even mental. To grasp their emergence from the void and their swirling confluence is to understand the very essence of nature and ourselves'.* So, how is this vast philosophy and mythology woven into the practice of ayurvedic medicine and its therapies? More importantly, what is it about ayurvedic medicine that may appeal to you and offer help?

Authoritative texts tell us that ayurvedic medicine originates from an oral tradition that organized the fundamentals of life into a system, what we know today as ayurveda. A word from Sanskrit, the ancient root language for most of Europe and Asia, ayurveda (I-your-vay-da) translates as 'science of life': *ayur* meaning life, and *veda* science or knowledge. This wisdom is at least 5,000 years old and handed down from the great seers of India, known as Rishis.

The core of ayurvedic medicine is the concept of three major *doshas*, known as *vata*, *pitta*, and *kapha*. Each *dosha* is a combined vital energy that reflects two of the five elements we find in tantric philosophy. *Vata* is a combination of air and ether, with air predominat-

*Ballentine, p. 181.

ing. *Pitta* combines fire and water, with fire predominant, and *kapha* combines water and earth, with water as the primary element. In ayurveda, the *doshas* and the state of their balance are responsible for all that goes on within us, both physically and psychologically. As in TCM, this balance affects how we relate internally to ourselves and externally to the environment around us. Ayurveda also teaches that we are born with a basic constitution that is determined by our individual configuration of *doshas*. Because we are talking about subtle energy, there are fine variations within each of us, which is what gives us our uniqueness.

We can think of our constitution as being a touchstone not only for our individuality but also as a measure for the state of balance of our health. While this concept may seem alien to the West, it really needn't be. If we pause to think about it, the idea of 'constitution' as it relates to health is not so unusual. In the Middle Ages, physicians routinely diagnosed a patient according to the major element of their constitution with words like sanguine, phlegmatic, or choleric. Referring to one's 'constitution' as a means of describing our robustness or otherwise is perfectly common today. 'Jonathan has the constitution of a horse.' 'I'm going out to take my constitutional.' However, although 'constitution' is familiar in this framework, the idea of a constitution in ayurvedic medicine has broader and far deeper implications, because of its relationship to the *doshas*.

Within our constitution, ayurveda says, one of the three *doshas* is predominant. Characteristics of the remaining two *doshas* are less predominant, although it sometimes happens that two of the three might be dominantly close in alignment. The ultimate goal in ayurveda is to help the individual maintain a state of balance between the three *doshas*, but more important is maintaining balance in the predominant *dosha* or *doshas*. Before delving into their characteristics, however, let us briefly look at who actually practises ayurvedic medicine.

YOUR AYURVEDIC PRACTITIONER

The qualifying degree in Ayurvedic Medicine and Surgery involves five years of extensive education and intense training from a recognized university or college that offers this course of study. Following the completion of these five years, the student must then enter into a period of supervised practice, similar to western medical internships. Practitioners of ayurvedic therapies, while not holding a degree in ayurvedic medicine and surgery, are nevertheless qualified through precise areas of training to advise and guide patients in various cleansing techniques, herbs, diet, and lifestyle changes.

At present, ayurvedic medicine is mainly practised in the West as preventative medicine, or as an approach in the treatment of certain chronic imbalances such as allergies, digestive disorders, auto-immune disorders and emotional illnesses, when western medicine has been ineffective. Thus, the medical challenges that ayurvedic physicians and practitioners face here are far less dramatic here than you would find in Southern Asia or Tibet, although this appears to be changing. Regardless of the situation, the ayurvedic physician or practitioner will approach you as patient from the perspective of wanting to know who you are. He or she wants to identify the configuration and state of balance of your *doshas*!

For a moment, let us suppose that you have been struggling with a chronic health situation that has progressively impacted the quality of your daily life. In an effort to return to a state of wellness, you have been to several medical specialists, each highly qualified in their field. Unfortunately, none of them can offer you any definitive answers and little substantive or permanent relief. Furthermore, during the course of your search you have also had extensive tests that are disappointingly unrevealing. As a last resort, you follow the advice of a friend who suggests you visit an ayurvedic physician. You arrive for your appointment with your records and films from the various examinations, feeling hopeful, only to be disappointed when the physician tells you that he or she is not particularly interested in looking at them. No doubt, you will find this shocking!

When we are feeling ill, western physicians will one way or another ask, 'How are you?'. This translates as, 'What are your symptoms?' On the other hand, an ayurvedic physician is interested in how you relate internally and externally to your environments, determined by the balance of your *doshas*. The very difference in these two approaches mirrors the root differences in how the physician assesses illness and how he or she has learned to practise medicine. The ayurvedic physician, like the practitioner of TCM, wants to know you through a myriad of questions that may seem like they have no relationship to illness or medicine.

Most likely, you will be asked to talk about the kinds of foods you like, whether spicy, bland, or sweet. What hours of the day, seasons, and climates, are your favourites? Which are your least favorites? How deeply do you sleep and how much? What are your relationships like, both personal and professional? What kind of work interests you? Do you exercise, and if so, what sort do you prefer? These questions are just a small sample of the areas the physician will be interested in, in an effort to build up an overall portrait of you. In the practitioner's mind, your answers to these questions are combined with his or her own observations. He or she might check your pulses (we have several), along with the condition of your skin and hair, and even note your body language. At this point, he or she will have a fairly constructive picture of your primary *dosha* type(s) and your constitution. Now you are ready to embark upon your 'holistic' path to vibrant health with expert advice to guide you.

WHAT IS YOUR *DOSHA*?

Now we can return to the individual characteristics of the *doshas*. It is important to keep in mind that assessment of your constitution by way of your *doshas* involves characteristics of physical build, physical distinctions, physiological functions, and psychological variables, all of which make up an individually complex picture. However, as a starting point, the chart opposite gives general characteristics of each of the *doshas*. It is important to keep in mind, however, that only a qualified physician or practitioner can make a comprehensively accurate evaluation.

Recalling that the goal of ayurveda is to keep you in balance in mind, body, and spirit, you will need to pay attention to the foods and activities that support this, and avoid those that may aggravate your *doshas*. Ayurveda notes a number of things that can affect them. These variables make for fascinating exploration through sources listed at the end of this book.

Meanwhile, to get you thinking within this frame-

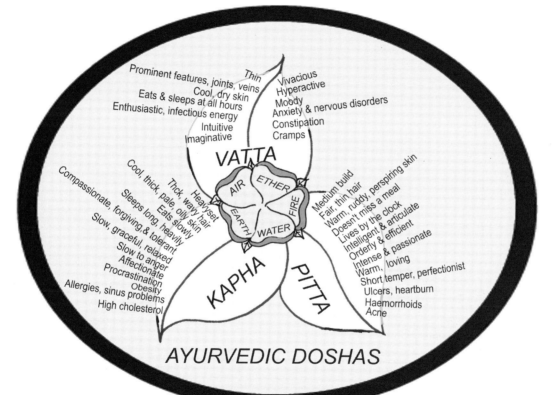

VATTA

Prominent features, joints, veins
Cool, dry skin
Eats & sleeps at all hours
Enthusiastic, infectious energy
Intuitive
Imaginative

Thin
Vivacious
Hyperactive
Moody
Anxiety & nervous disorders
Constipation
Cramps

AIR ETHER
EARTH FIRE
WATER

KAPHA

Compassionate, forgiving,& tolerant
Cool, thick, pale, oily skin
Thick, wavy hair
Heavyset
Sleeps long, heavily
Eats slowly
Slow, graceful, relaxed
Slow to anger
Affectionate
Procrastination
Obesity
Allergies, sinus problems
High cholesterol

PITTA

Medium build
Fair, thin hair
Warm, ruddy, perspiring skin
Doesn't miss a meal
Lives by the clock
Intelligent & articulate
Orderly & efficient
Intense & passionate
Warm, loving
Short temper, perfectionist
Ulcers, heartburn
Haemorrhoids
Acne

AYURVEDIC DOSHAS

CHARACTERISTICS
OF AYURVEDIC BODYTYPES

work, let us consider from the ayurvedic viewpoint where there is potential for illness to develop. To an ayurvedic physician or practitioner, our lifestyle—and how we respond to it—is a vital element, along with our physiological processes of intake, digestion, and elimination. Much of what happens to us as it relates to a state of health is dependent on our internal and external environments by way of our digestive and excretory tracts.

Proper digestion and elimination of *ama* is a critical cornerstone of ayurveda. *Ama* is a collection of toxic substances that the body disposes of when digestion is functioning properly. However, if digestion is weak because the 'fire' of the *pitta dosha* is lacking, *ama* will build up in various parts of the body, thereby blocking the channels through which subtle energy, *prana* (*qi* in TCM) flows. In Chapter Three, we learned that in TCM, blockage of the flow of *qi* along the meridians weakens the body, creating an opening for illness. In ayurveda, the build-up of *ama* is considered 'a major cause of illness'.* Engaging in non-beneficial lifestyle activities, along with a diet that is in conflict with our primary *dosha*(s) will make it hard for our system to digest food properly, or to assimilate necessary nutrients and eliminate *ama*.

If our system is lacking in necessary nutrients, and

*Morrison, THE BOOK OF AYURVEDA, p. 77.

lacks the ability to eliminate harmful toxins, our central nervous system will be affected. In turn, if this is compromised, our ability to handle day-to-day stressors will be impaired. Stress factors in our daily life that were once hardly noticeable now become major. Our doshic levels and constitutional balance have now become what practitioners call 'aggravated', meaning out of balance. When this happens, we need to engage in activities and eat foods that are 'pacifying' to our primary *dosha* or *doshas*, facilitating the disposal of the *ama*, so that we may enter into a state of strength and balance. Clearly, if we remain in a state of doshic imbalance, we are setting ourselves up for the emergence of illness.

It is important to point out that inappropriate lifestyles and diet are not the only factors that can affect our constitutional balance. Life-events such as trauma, loss, surgery, and extreme stress or anxiety, can also affect it. Another aspect to consider is that in these situations we have the perfect opportunity to take advantage of 'integrative medicine'. As with many of the therapies we are dealing with, Ayurveda can beautifully support us in medical situations that initially require the skill and technology of western medicine, such as emergency trauma or surgery. By embracing those things in our recovery that support our *doshas*, we have an opportunity of perhaps shortening the timeline of fully recovering our balance and strength.

A PLAN FOR YOU

As I mentioned earlier in this chapter, the ayurvedic physician or qualified practitioner will suggest a plan or protocol that is specifically for you. The guidelines it sets down are for the sole purpose of supporting (or, if necessary, strengthening and pacifying) your *doshas*. Such a plan typically includes suggestions for appropriate foods, types of activity that are beneficial, and relaxation techniques such as breathing exercises, meditation, and yoga postures. In addition, your practitioner will also discuss those things you need to avoid as they can aggravate your primary *dosha(s)*.*

Ayurvedic physicians and practitioners also incorporate specific herbs and cleansing techniques that are unique to ayurveda. Ayurvedic herbs are used for pacification, rejuvenation and maintenance, and are often in the form of capsules or teas.

Panchakarma refers to distinctive cleansing techniques used in ayurveda. The procedures of *panchakarma* are not therapies that a physician or practitioner will suggest frivolously. Thus, only a qualified ayurvedic physician or practitioner should administer or supervise them. *Panchakarma* translates as 'five actions'. These actions are means of deep cleansing in order to rid the body of excess *dosha* elements and toxins. They include, 'therapeutic vomiting to remove excess *pitta* [fire], therapeutic enema to remove excess *vata* [air], nasal [wash] in cases of diseases of the head and neck, and bloodletting in cases of blood disorders'.*

While *panchakarma* may sound dramatic, scary and even medieval (bloodletting!), it is important to keep in mind that these therapies are called upon in a very judicious manner by the practitioner. In most cases, there may be a period of preparation, involving the use of herbs and oil massage in advance of the cleansing. Furthermore, there are also techniques you can use on your own, as in the case of a very simple (and painless) nasal wash should you develop nasal congestion or sinus blockage. The nasal wash is also an excellent preventive care therapy, should you be susceptible to chronic colds and sinus difficulties.

In considering the choice between traditional Chinese medicine and ayurveda for your healing journey, it is important to keep in mind that one is not better than the other. The reality is that your decision will come down to personal comfort and faith in the tradition's methodology and philosophy, and, of course, the availability of a qualified practitioner. In any case, both traditions prompt changes in lifestyle and perspectives that are significant to attaining internal

*Useful breathing exercises are given in Jenny Beeken's DON'T HOLD YOUR BREATH (Polair, 2004, uniform with the present book),

*Morrison, p. 186.

and external harmony and balance. This is important to your awareness, for if you were in harmony and balance, it is unlikely you would be seeking out complementary healthcare options.

Although not as abundant in America as in Great Britain, there are several good ayurvedic cookbooks and restaurants available that can give you a 'taste' of ayurveda's approach to nutrition.

In closing this chapter, we also need to be reminded that ayurveda additionally draws upon therapies that are not exclusive to its tradition, including yoga, breathing techniques, and meditation. The remedies of homeopathy and cell or tissue salts are often used in ayurveda as well, to which we now turn as we travel from East to West, in Chapter Five.

CHAPTER FOUR KEY POINTS:

- Ayurveda, like TCM, is a complete system of medicine, and approximately 5,000 years old.
- Ayurveda seeks to balance body, mind and spirit through the three main centres of vital energy, *doshas*. The *doshas* are identified by their predominant element: *vata* (air), *pitta* (fire) and *kapha* (water)
- Each individual has one prominent *dosha*, or possibly two *doshas* that share predominance.
- Aggravation of *doshas* is a result of excess *dosha* elements and toxins (*ama*) that have accumulated in the body through inappropriate diet and lifestyle.
- Pacification of *doshas* involves 'burning off' excess *dosha* elements and *ama* through correction in diet, lifestyle, herbs, and cleansing therapies.
- Ayurvedic philosophy and therapies can be adopted in small steps, a few at a time.

CHAPTER FIVE

LIKE CURES LIKE:

THE MYSTERIES OF HOMEOPATHY

IF WE wanted to identify the complementary therapy that most continuously sparks controversy with allopathic medicine, it probably would be homeopathy. Traditionally, the practice of homeopathy has been more widely accepted in Europe than in the USA. While homeopathy has chronically been under attack by the American medical establishment, the degree of intensity has not always been at the current level. For all this, homeopathy has a multifaceted history that goes back more than two hundred years; and interestingly enough, despite the intensely rekindled efforts to discredit it, it continues to experience a remarkable rejuvenation.

The three things most important in homeopathy are its 'remedies', its principle of the body having the ability to heal from within (given the stimulus to do so); and, most importantly, its recognition of the unique characteristics an illness presents within each individual. It thus shares many things with the eastern medical systems, but the principle of healing from within is a major

contribution to the thought-system of complementary therapies, and recurs in the subtle therapies with which later chapters deal. Another homeopathic principle is 'like cures like'. This perspective is in marked conflict with Newtonian physics. It also conflicts with educated logic, the foundations of modern drug therapy and the biomedical model of medicine.

For its conception, homeopathy credits a German physician, Samuel Hahnemann (1755–1843). He had become disillusioned with the manner in which his colleagues were practising. The cause of his distress lay with many of the commonly-accepted treatments that, to Hahnemann, rendered the patient more harm than benefit. In the course of translating William Cullen's TREATISE OF THE MATERIA MEDICA into German, Hahnemann became intrigued with what Cullen had to say about the use of cinchona bark in the treatment of malaria. Hahnemann discounted Cullen's claim that the bark possessed 'stomach-strengthening properties'. He took it upon himself to disprove this claim by ingesting 'four drams of Peruvian bark twice daily for several days to attempt to characterize the action of the quinine-containing bark'.*

To his amazement, Hahnemann found that the bark produced the intermittent fevers common to malaria. This result led him to speculate that if an otherwise healthy individual developed side-effects by ingesting a specific medical substance, these could provide a useful guideline to a specific substance's healing properties.†Hahnemann's experiment thus led to the revolutionary theory of 'like cures like'. Moving forward, he took his research through strenuous tests (known as 'provings') of numerous substances on healthy individuals. As he had speculated, these identified the effectiveness of specific substances in treating precise symptoms in illness.

Hahnemann further discovered that in treatment, doses producing extreme symptoms were inappropriate. This led him to deduce that by reducing dosages to infinitesimal levels, through successive dilutions of first tenfold and then a hundredfold, their 'potency' or effect, increased. Today, this method is known as the homeopathic 'Law of the Infinitesimal Dose'.

If Hahnemann's theories on the treatment of illness were viewed as eccentric to colleagues at the time, his views on its causes were most likely even more so.

From the outset, it appears that Hahnemann's views on why we become ill were of a spiritual nature. 'In the healthy condition of man, the spiritual vital force (autocracy), the dynamis that animates the material body (organism), rules with unbounded sway.... Without the vital force, [the body] is capable of no sensation, no function, no self-preservation', he wrote.*

Without wanting to stretch the point too far, I suggest that Hahnemann's beliefs about the cause of illness closely relate to the philosophies found in traditional Chinese medicine and ayurveda: that is, a disturbance in one's vital life-force (qi, prana) is an opportunity for illness. Hahnemann and his theories remind us, yet again, that our state of wellness is a mirror of environments and landscapes within and without.

Fortunately, Hahnemann's theories did not die with his passing. Research continued, and still continues, so that today there are thousands of homeopathic remedies in existence. They are made from natural substances such as plants, minerals, and animals, rendering homeopathy a powerful integrative therapy which can be used alongside western medicine or complete systems of healing such as traditional Chinese medicine and ayurveda. Additionally, its repertoire of remedies is one that has evolved substantially.

Sadly, because homeopathy is one more therapy

*http://altmed.creighton.edu/Homeopathy/history.htm.
†Gerber, VIBRATIONAL MEDICINE, p. 115.

*http://altmed.creighton.edu/Homepathy/philosophy/cause.htm

not conducive to the research parameters demanded by western science, it continues to struggle for a place of widespread acceptance as a significant, integrative therapy in eyes of the western medical establishment. This is despite a great deal of recognition in certain quarters. 'The World Health Organization has cited homeopathy as one of the systems of traditional medicine that should be integrated worldwide with conventional medicine in order to provide adequate global healthcare in the twenty-first century', says one publication. 'In Britain, homeopathic hospitals and outpatient clinics are part of the national health system, and homeopathy is recognized as a postgraduate medical specialty by virtue of an act of Parliament.'*

However, conflict between medical theories is not the complete story. As is often the case with the herbal remedies of traditional Chinese medicine and ayurveda, homeopathic remedies are relatively inexpensive. The economic differences between the medicines of modern allopathy and complementary therapies therefore present another area of conflict, although it is not one that usually publicly debated. Interestingly, this issue of economics is one that is far from being recent. According to Richard Gerber, MD, author of VIBRATIONAL MEDICINE FOR THE TWENTY-FIRST CENTURY, 'Few laypeople are aware that the burgeoning homeopathic movement was one of the driving forces behind the formation of the American Medical Association (AMA). The non-homeopathic or "allopathic" physicians who used drugs and surgery as their only form of treatment believed that there was an encroachment of homeopaths upon what was considered the allopathic physician's "economic turf". The political pressure exerted by MDs to fight homeopathy back in the 1800s was so vehement that one of the early bylaws of the AMA included a section strictly prohibiting fraternization with homeopathic practitioners or medicinal use of homeopathic remedies.'*

Even in Hahnemann's time political and economic turf wars were active, as he unashamedly points out: 'For several centuries, a whole range of causes … have led to the downgrading of that divine science, clinical medicine, to the level of a wretched, money-grubbing exercise in the whitewashing of symptoms and a demeaning traffic in prescriptions.'†

HOW THE REMEDIES ARE MADE

Leaving history, turf wars and economics behind, we now need to understand how homeopathy works, and how it can help you. For a beginning let us turn to the

*Trivieri and Anderson, pp. 270–1.

*Gerber, p. 115.
†http://altmed.creighton.edu/homeopathy/quotes.htm.

father of American homeopathy, Dr Constantine Hering, who stated in the mid-nineteenth century, 'Healing progresses from the deepest part of the body to the extremities; from the emotional and mental aspects to the physical; from the upper part of the body … to the lower parts of the body.… [Furthermore,] healing progresses in reverse chronological order, from the most recent maladies to the oldest'.* In contemplating this, it helps to have the image of the opening of a flower. The outer petals open first—or, in the case of illness, the least bothersome effects of illness are healed (or balanced) first, revealing the deeper roots of the illness.

There is another reason for many allopathic physicians to write off homeopathy's successes as coincidence, or a result of the 'placebo effect'.† Despite various plausible theories, we still have no conclusive evidence to explain how or why it works. There is recent speculation however, that the answer to these questions may lie in the field of quantum physics.‡ If this proves to be true, even the most stringent critics will find it difficult to continue in their scepticism.

In the meantime, 'potentization' (the unique method used to prepare homeopathic remedies) makes acceptance difficult by rational, scientific minds. Homeopathic remedies differ from other forms of medicine in that they straddle the worlds of physical and energetic or vibrational medicine (a concept we shall discuss shortly). The intention behind homeopathic remedies is that they are used to balance out dysfunction by stimulating the body's own ability to heal from within. This is somewhat similar to the philosophy behind the allopathic treatment of allergies, and vaccines. However, how a homeopathic remedy affects our physical, emotional, and perhaps spiritual level at any given time largely depends upon the potency prescribed and the sought-after result.

As we saw, Hahnemann discovered that by diluting the dose of a normally toxic substance to an infinitesimal amount, the substance could be proved effective in treating specific illnesses. Thus, the more a substance was diluted, the greater the power of its healing effect! For most of us, understanding details of the dilution process involved in the production of homeopathic remedies is a mathematical maze. It is not necessary to grasp these details in order to benefit from the remedies. Having said this, for readers who possess insatiable curiosity, a simplified example of the dilution process is given opposite.

For the average individual, the important point about potencies in homeopathic remedies is that the

*Trivieri and Anderson, p. 273.

†The 'placebo effect' is a term often used in medicine that refers to a measurable, observable, or felt improvement in health not attributable to treatment, but often with psychological implications.

‡Trivieri and Anderson, p. 272.

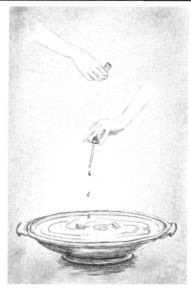

THE PREPARATION OF AN "X" POTENCY HOMEOPATHIC REMEDY

1. Plant such as healing herb, mineral or animal substance placed in mixture of alcohol and water.

2. Infused material is thoroughly ground up and filtered.

3. Filtered liquid = 'mother tincture'.

4. 1 drop of mother tincture is added to 9 drops of water = 1:10 dilution ('X' potency).

5. Mixture is rapidly 'succussed'* or shaken.

6. Following 'succussion' of the 1X (1:10 dilution) remedy, 1 drop of this remedy is then added to another 9 drops of water + succussion = 2X (1:10) remedy.

Thus the process continues, providing a repertoire of remedies ranging from potencies wherein a dilution of one part mother tincture to nine drops of water yields an 'X' potency remedy, to extremely high dilutions where there is no measurable chemical trace of material in the remedy.

*'Succussion' is a term native to the creation of homeopathic remedies. The dilution containing the 'mother tincture' is rapidly shaken in order to stimulate the energy of the remedy.

number before a potency indicates how many times the solution has been progressively diluted, i.e., a '6X' potency has been diluted six times using one part substance from the preceding solution to nine parts water formula. The description of a potency as '1C' tells us that one drop of mother tincture has been diluted with ninety-nine drops of water (1:100) and a '1M' potency would indicate one drop of mother tincture has been added to 999 drops of water (1:1000) and so on. Common potencies available in mass-market pharmacies are, 6X, 12X, 30X, 6C, 12C, 30C and sometimes 200C.

These work on the material level of the physical

body, although the 200Cs are believed to work on the energetic levels as well.* The higher potencies, such as 1M, 10M and those even higher, have been diluted so many times that these remedies containing no chemical trace of material and are considered to function at a higher energetic level or 'vibration'. When we recall that healing through homeopathy works from the inside out, it may be obvious that these deeper remedies work with the subtle energy layers of our body, particularly those having to do with deeply-buried, toxic emotions, such as repressed anger or grief. Additionally, in cases of trauma or emotional distress, whether old or more recent, these particular remedies can be extremely powerful healing tools. As human beings, we carry the memories of trauma deep within us: they are significant parts of our personal history. Repressed emotions and memories of trauma alike are catalysts for illness if not resolved.

The higher potencies are usually available only through homeopathic chemists (or pharmacies), or homeopathic practitioners. In this case, it is unlikely that a reputable homeopathic chemist or pharmacy would sell them to an individual without thorough inquiry as to the intended use and the individual's knowledge of homeopathy, for obvious reasons. It is extremely

*200C actually is a borderline between working on both the physical and emotional, depending on the situation.

important to remember that some homeopathic remedies are dilutions of substances that can be dangerously toxic or poisonous. In the lower potencies (from the homeopathic point of view) this is not an issue of concern. However if the high-potency remedies are misused, there can be serious consequences, as with all drugs. For similar reasons, and as with traditional Chinese medicine and ayurveda, it is wise to investigate carefully the qualifications of either the pharmacist or the practitioner from whom you are seeking guidance.

One of the advantages of homeopathy is that the lower potencies, such as those in the 'X', and the lower C ranges, prepared with fewer dilutions, safely address physical symptoms and minor illnesses, and can be called upon for treating simple, everyday ailments. Examples include colds, flu, symptoms of allergies, or light-to-moderate anxiety in both children and adults.

SCHUESSLER SALTS

Before turning to the subject of what to expect when working with a homeopathic practitioner, it is important to briefly mention the subject of 'cell salts', also known as tissue salts or Schuessler salts, as they are often prescribed in conjunction with a homeopathic course of treatment. At the end of the nineteenth century, Cell salts were discovered by another German physician,

Wilhelm Heinrich Schuessler. Similar to homeopathic remedies, they function on the material level, but can also have a subtle effect at the psychological level too.

Schuessler's research focused on the twelve essential minerals that are already present in our tissues. He believed that if there were a deficiency in these minerals, the imbalance would lead to health problems. He further theorized that by supplementing the body in these deficiencies, restoration of the body's mineral balance was possible. Keeping in mind that Schuessler's twelve salts are compounds already present in the body, we are told that their supplementation purpose is to act as catalysts by 'reorganizing the tissue functions, lifting those tissues out of the pattern of dysfunction so that they begin to function properly'.*

Tissue salts are similar to homeopathic remedies, but far less complicated in preparation. Essentially a compound of one part mineral to nine parts lactose is ground up (now by mechanical means), just as one would have done in the old days with a mortar and pestle. After approximately one hour of grinding, the resulting potency is a 1X. To create a 6X potency, the 1X is ground again with another nine parts lactose, the process being repeated six times. The concept behind the repeated grinding is that with each successive grinding the closer one is to the pure essence of the salt.†

*Ballentine, p. 54. †Ballentine, p. 53.

Today the repertoire of tissue salts remains at Schuessler's original twelve (though combinations are on the market also), and abbreviations of the Latin names of the salts are used: Calc Flor (Calcium Fluoride), Calc Phos (Calcium Phosphate), Calc Sulph (Calcium Sulphate), Ferr Phos (Ferric Phosphate), Kali Mur (Potassium Chloride), Kali Phos (Potassium Phosphate), Kali Sulph (Potassium Sulphate), Mag Phos (Magnesium Phosphate), Nat Mur (Sodium Chloride), Nat Phos (Sodium Phosphate), Nat Sulph (Sodium Sulphate) and Silica (Silicic acid/Silica).

A VISIT TO A HOMEOPATH

Let us now look at what you can expect if you visit a homeopathic practitioner, at how the remedies and salts are used by a homeopathic practitioner, and how they can be useful as part of your home medicine kit.

In choosing a homeopathic practitioner, you should research his or her background and credentials just as you would any other practitioner in complementary medicine. You may find that your homeopath is also an MD, but this is not always the case, nor is it essential. Credentials identifying qualified homeopathic practitioners differ between the United States and Great Britain and thus it would be wise to contact either National Center for Homeopathy in the U.S., or the British

Homeopathic Association, when seeking a referral. You will find contact information for both of these organizations under 'Further Resources' at the end of this book.

Consultation with a homeopath does not differ a great deal from the process you meet when consulting a practitioner of traditional Chinese medicine or ayurveda. The homeopath will take a complete history that is similar in many ways to the processes described in the other traditions. And, as in those situations, you will be asked to describe any symptoms that you are currently experiencing, including any emotional distress you may be under. It is important to understand that homeopathy is not an invasive medicine, and that it is based in its remedies (and in some cases, Schuessler's tissue salts).

Depending on your diagnosis, the Homeopath may at first prescribe some lower-potency remedies to address symptoms that are the most evident or bothersome to you. As these balance out, the more deeply-rooted issues will become evident and thus, available for harmonization (remember the image of the flower given earlier). As you progress through your course of treatment, he or she then may prescribe one or more 'constitutional powders' (see below, no. 3). These are the remedies that are the higher dilutions or potencies, and are the ones that work on the subtle energy layers of our body. Remember, in the philosophy of alternative medicine, it is these deeper emotions that can be very toxic to our wellbeing, and thus are the driving force behind chronic illness.

While tissue salts come in one form only, homeopathic remedies come in several, all of which are tasteless. They are taken under the tongue, where they dissolve quite quickly. The forms are typically lactose-based and are as follows.

1. Globs: tiny white round pills (these can be either low or high potencies).

2. Small soluble tablets (Schuessler's tissue salts are such as these).

3. Powders: usually but not always the higher-potency remedies such as a '1M', known as 'constitutionals', prescribed to address imbalances in your basic 'constitution', similar to the concept as used in TCM and ayurveda.

4. Mixes: usually one or two tissue salts ground together to form a powder mixture.

5. Liquid tinctures (low potencies).

There are several essential guidelines to follow when on a course of homeopathic treatments, some of which are listed below:

• Homeopathic remedies are never touched with your fingers, as any residue on them can interfere with the potency of the remedy.

• When taking a homeopathic remedy, do not have food in your mouth.

• It is inadvisable to drink coffee, use minted toothpaste, or ingest other strong-tasting substances, as these also can interfere with the remedy's effectiveness.

Your practitioner will instruct you on how to incorporate these powerful healing tools into your life and most likely will offer helpful lifestyle suggestions too.

Homeopathy integrates very easily with allopathic medicine, especially as a support if you are recovering from something that required crisis intervention.

In addition to prescribing remedies, cell salts, and lifestyle-change suggestions such as alterations in diet, your Homeopath may also suggest flower remedies. These were discovered in the 1920s by the British physician, Edward Bach. Like tissue salts, flower essences are homeopathic in nature, but function quite differently from the remedies we have explored so far, and it is to Bach's work that we shall now look.

CHAPTER FIVE KEY POINTS:

1. Homeopathy has a history going back two hundred years.

2. It is recognized as a major therapy in Europe and countries such as India. It does not currently enjoy the same status in America, although this seems to be slowly changing.

3. Homeopathy's major philosophy is 'like cures like', and this forms the foundation for its remedies. They stimulate the body's own ability to heal.

4. Depending on potency, homeopathic remedies address imbalances on different levels: physical, emotional, and possibly spiritual.

5. Homeopathy is non-invasive and is a safe therapy for both children and adults, although the higher-potency remedies should be used under the supervision of a qualified practitioner.

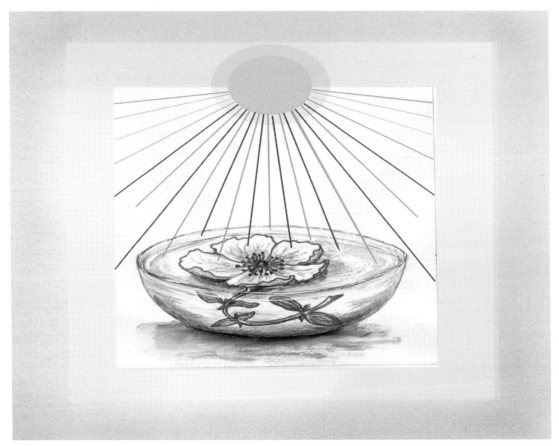

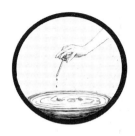

CHAPTER SIX

THE BACH FLOWER REMEDIES:

THE GREAT COMMUNICATORS BETWEEN SPIRIT, MIND AND BODY

THE THEME that recurs across the whole breadth of complementary medicine is that nature's abundance provides tools to help us in our efforts to achieve balance in body, mind, and spirit. In the preceding chapters, we have had glimpses of the ways in which traditional Chinese medicine and ayurveda call upon nature's herbs for healing. In Chapter Five, we learned that homeopathy utilizes what the animal, plant, and mineral kingdoms can offer in the creation of its remedies.

Therapies such as these straddle a divide between the words of physical and vibrational medicine or 'energetic' medicine. Yet while the therapies used in TCM, ayurveda, and homeopathy are 'vibrational' in nature, there are therapies that are considered to be exclusively vibrational medicine. This is because they do not contain any significantly measurable chemical or physical material in their remedies or in any other aspect of the therapy or practice. Instead, they focus

on balancing dysfunctions that exist within the subtle layers of energy that surround our body as well as the internal energetic environment of our emotions. It is in this realm of exclusive vibrational therapies, that we encounter Edward Bach's thirty-eight famous Flower Remedies.*

Edward Bach was a highly-respected British physician, with a reputation built upon his expertise in the fields of bacteriology, immunology and pathology. In the later 1920s, he began to experience frustration and disappointment in the way that medicine was not

*The word 'remedies' is used worldwide to describe Bach's preparations and those of people who have followed in his footsteps. However in the US, the Federal Food & Drug Administration prohibits us from using this word in connection to Dr Bach's work. Thus, they are known in the US as 'flower essences'. However, I have chosen to honour Dr Bach's original terminology and therefore will continue to use 'flower remedies' throughout this book; in spite of the FDA.

treating the 'whole person'. Bach shared this with Hahnemann, whose theories he had been studying.

Although Bach's medical education had been a traditional one, there was a spirituality that went with it, and recognition of what a healer was in the wider sense. From youth, he 'knew' that he was meant to be a healer; it was simply a matter of whether he would practise this vocation through the ministry or through medicine. Fortunately for all of us, he chose medicine.

From early on, the orthodox medical community considered Bach a genius in his chosen specialities. He had a large research laboratory in London in addition to a consulting practice in Harley Street.* While his work as an orthodox physician was highly regarded, his work in bacteriology and homeopathy gained him considerable reputations as well, some aspects of which are still recognized today. In addition, Bach possessed a gift of heightened intuition that dictated how he practised as a physician throughout his career. In the course of treating his patients, he became aware of a connection between their emotional states of mind and their chronic symptoms. This observation led him to develop theories on illness not unlike those associated with Hippocrates and Hahnemann.

*For readers in America, Chicago's Michigan Avenue or New York's Park Avenue physicians enjoy status comparable to London's Harley Street medical consultants, even today.

Illness, he believed, was a result of a disharmony between our intended life-path as mandated by our individual soul and personality. Furthermore, he believed that if this disconnection were not harmonized, the body eventually would break down. Here again we see the common thread that runs through the philosophy of complementary medicine and its therapies.

Overall, it is important to keep in mind that Bach placed importance in the relationship between emotions and illness, and the need for each of us to recognize our own spiritual divinity. Thus for him, balancing distressed emotions and spiritual health were equal keys to wellness.

As an individual, Bach found it difficult to function in the busy London environment—understandable, given his intuitive sensitivity. Personal balance could be found in nature, whether it was walking the quiet parks of London or having the opportunity to wander the fields and lanes of the English countryside. For Bach, nature held the answer to the difficulties we face in life because it brings balance in body, mind, and spirit. He believed that in this life as a physician his 'soul path' was to find nature's solution to harmonizing the disharmonious emotions that underlay illness and disease.

Whether it was science, his heightened intuitive abilities, or a combination of the two that led to his early experiments in nature, we simply do not know.

His longtime assistant, Nora Weeks (who wrote a great deal about Bach's work after his death), does not reveal these details to us in her writings. Perhaps even she did not know for certain, as there was a very private side of Bach that apparently was not even available to her.

What we do know is that around 1928 Bach had been experimenting with oral vaccines in his immunological research; and that it was also in 1928 that he prepared his first flower remedies using a similar method to the preparation of oral vaccines. These first remedies were prepared from specific species of the flowers mimulus, clematis and impatiens. Upon administration to some of his patients for particular distressed emotional states, they showed results way beyond his wildest expectations. Thus he knew he had discovered something important. In 1930, he left London and orthodox medicine behind, in order to expand his focus on this discovery.

By taking his work in bacteriology and homeopathy out of the lab and into nature, Bach recognized that there was a delicate energetic and spiritual relationship between the subtle life-force (*qi, prana*) of certain flowers and human emotions. Those who knew him have written that as his intuition became heightened, he could hold a petal or leaf from a flower or plant and accurately 'intuit' its healing ability. Moreover, toward the end of his life, Bach was simply able to hold his hand over a plant in order to know its healing potential.

It is important to recognize that at the heart of the Bach Flower Remedies is a spiritual and energetic energy. The healing energy or 'vibration' (a word that Bach himself used) within each of his chosen flowers is capable of balancing distressed emotional states that occur within each of us as human beings.

Bach died at the early age of 50 in 1936, but seventy years on his remedies are globally known and used. Considered homeopathic in nature and functioning in the realm of vibrational or energy medicine, at least another forty major flower essence repertoires now exist worldwide, all of them based on Dr Bach's work. In this remarkable evolution, the remedies have fuelled a radical shift in some circles regarding the manner in which distressed emotions and illnesses are treated.

If Bach were physically with us today, he would no doubt be astonished at the global spread of his work in the last seventy or so years. In addition to the major flower remedy repertoires, there are thousands of individuals who prepare their own flower remedies from their gardens and the fields of nature—as Bach himself encouraged people to do. Yet the fact that the discovery of flower-remedy therapy is universally acknowledged as his speaks for the brilliance of Bach's work.

With such expansion of his work have come many excellent resources to guide people throughout the world. They are examining his discoveries, studying his guidelines, and using the formulas and remedies in their daily lives. Several of these resources are listed in the 'Further Reading' section at the end of this book.

WHY DO THEY WORK?

We now need to examine why and how flower remedies can help us in our healing process. As it was Bach's belief that conflict between the soul's agenda and the personality resulted in illness, he was explicit in his opinion that each of the thirty-eight remedies possessed a specific energetic and emotional signature. Furthermore, he was convinced that these signatures were capable of balancing out negative or contracted emotional states that clouded the soul's innate wisdom.

Bach's philosophy extended to the point of saying that when we move into an emotional state that is distressed, it is as if a fog or cloud drops over this wisdom, so that we are no longer able to 'see' clearly. This represents the very foundation of how Bach believed the remedies worked. They are all about perception. If our wisdom is fogged over, so is our perception of our external environment. This perception affects how we internally interpret this environment, prompting a positive or negative response. Bach felt that the life-force, the energy, *qi* or *prana*, in each of the specific flowers,

had the capability to lift the fog, resulting in perception-shifts to a more realistic picture and interpretation.

In 1935, with the identification of thirty-eight negative emotions and the precise flower remedies that were effective in addressing them, Bach announced that his work was finished, The common emotions of fear, anger, shame, guilt, mild to moderate depression, jealousy, rage, self-pity, and grief are among those that Bach focused on. While Bach's basic system of healing is limited to thirty-eight remedies, it is important to mention that there are actually more than two hundred million possible combinations of the thirty-eight. Even the most determined hypochondriac will have no fear of running out of remedy possibilities! Moreover, we can think of the thirty-eight like the colour spectrum: within each basic colour, there are hundreds of subtle variations. This is because the remedies can and do work simultaneously on various levels within us, whether the temporal (temporary), the thematic emotional (those emotions that are part of our whole history), and the spiritual. Every emotion has a range and every emotion has drivers that also range in subtlety.

In the early years of his work, Bach fine-tuned the system, changing the selection of flowers as well as changing his mind on which emotions needed to be addressed. His choices were based on observations of his patients, himself, and those around him. In the latter stages of his work, many of his selections were based on personal emotional states, which could be extreme.

It is useful now to explain how the remedies were and still are produced, according to Dr Bach's instructions, by the Bach Centre and also by Healing Herbs, Ltd. To begin with, only the blooms, and in some cases, the stems and leaves from the selected species, are used. They are harvested at the height of blossoming, as Bach believed it was the blossom of the flower that held the strongest healing energy of the plant. The flowers are placed in glass or crystal bowls filled with spring water. Left in the sunshine for approximately three hours, the flowers are then removed from the water by use of other plant material.* To the remaining water, an equal part of brandy is added as a preservative. This resulting mixture is the 'mother tincture'.† In order to make the small remedy bottles sold to the public, drops from the preserved mother tincture are further diluted in spring water and brandy in order to produce the small bottles that are available for purchase.*

The remedies are perfectly safe for use throughout one's lifetime. There are no contra-indications with other therapies or medications that you may be taking (unless you are alcohol-sensitive), or concern that you might become desensitized to them. If you do not wish to take the remedies by mouth, they can be effectively used in other ways: for example, on the pulse points, in the bath, or in massage oils. As human beings, our emotions are in constant flux. As they are ever-changing, we can continually call upon the remedies, one after another, throughout our lifetime. In addition, they can be safely used by adults and children as well as on animals and plants.

Sceptics often draw on the placebo theory to discount the effectiveness of the remedies. However, because they readily work on children (including infants) and animals, this theory does not hold water. Indeed, children, infants, and animals tend to respond more quickly to the remedies, as they have not had a lifetime to build up the protective emotional armour that we adults tend to create.

Of all the therapies we've explored here, flower-

*This procedure applies to approximately half of the repertoire; for the remaining remedies, the flowers are boiled for approximately thirty minutes on top of a stove and then left to cool. The only difference between the two methods is the source of heat. There is speculation as to why Bach chose the two differing methods, but no conclusive answer.

†The mother tinctures for the 'Original Bach Flower Remedies' are still made today at the Bach Centre by Trustees of the Dr Edward Bach Foundation according to Dr Bach's instructions.

*Additional information on preparation and personal application can be found in several of the references listed under 'Further Resources'.

remedy therapy in general is the one that is most suitable for self-help. However, while there is substantial literature to guide you in self-administration of the remedies (of which up to seven can be used in combination), there are occasions when a more extensive evaluation is called for through the expertise of a qualified flower remedy practitioner. One of the largest referral networks available is through the Dr Edward Bach Centre in England (details in 'Resources'). In addition, complementary practitioners who are qualified in other therapies may also be proficient in the field of flower remedies. This is especially true if they have a background in psychology. However, as with choosing a practitioner in all complementary therapies, it is equally wise to research the primary source of the remedy repertoire with which you wish to work, and its methods.

As to why flower remedies work, there is no clear answer. They are homeopathic in character, but not considered 'classical homeopathy' for reasons too extensive for this discussion. However, flower remedies as a complementary therapy are predisposed to the same mysteries as to why and how the high potencies of homeopathy work. In fact, some complementary physicians feel that flower remedies in general function at a higher vibratory level than the highest potencies of homeopathic remedies, yet they are extremely gentle.

As with all holistic therapies, the remedies are a system of healing that involves participation, awareness, reflection, and growth. It is important to understand that they can take us down to our core, and that this journey is a distinct process. It is one that requires examination of our emotional self within the framework of our external world and personal history. In this process, the remedies gently meet us wherever we are emotionally. They begin by bringing to our attention the emotions that are most bothersome, so that we may take action by addressing them. Then, layer by layer, they act as catalysts, facilitating transformation of repetitive patterns that are toxic for us. Moving our personal mythology from darkness to light, they break up the soil that holds the roots of negative emotions. In this way, they shift the perceptions within our emotional environment from fantasy to reality.

Furthermore, the remedies are as unobtrusive as working with the breath. They are agents of change; they are all about harmonizing emotional discord within us in order to prevent the development of illness and disease. In order to take full advantage of them, we have to explore where we become emotionally stuck and why. Sometimes this exploration requires assistance and/or support from other types of therapies, such as various forms of psychotherapy or spiritual advice. In such situations, the remedies can be a beautiful adjunct to personal work. While this exploration may be a difficult one, it's as if they provide a safe space for us while we examine this internal territory. In this space, we may take responsibility for our own wellbeing.

Taking responsibility for our own wellness (however difficult that may be to achieve) is something that Bach believed was necessary in order for us to manifest our highest good in this lifetime. As he himself said, 'Those Herbs of the field placed for Healing, by comforting, by soothing, by relieving our cares, our anxieties [bring] us nearer to the Divinity within. And it is that increase of the Divinity within which heals us…. Thus we can truly say that certain Herbs have been placed for us by Divine means, and the help which they give to us, not only heals our bodies, but brings into our lives, our characters, attributes of our Divinity.'*

*Masonic Lecture, Wallingford, UK, October 1936. Howard & Ramsell, p. 44. For further insight into Bach's spiritual philosophy, see IGNITING SOUL FIRE, listed in 'Further Reading'.

CHAPTER SIX KEY POINTS:

1. Bach believed that illness and disease is a result of conflict between the personality and our soul's plan for this lifetime.
2. Flower remedies are homeopathic in nature, using the blossoms of non-poisonous flowers and trees.
3. They work directly to harmonize our negative emotions.
4. They work equally on emotions that are temporary and long-term, and also on those that prevent soul growth.
5. They can be safely used throughout one's lifetime.
6. They are safe for adults, children, animals and plants, and they are not a placebo.

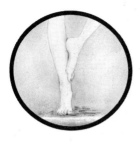

CHAPTER SEVEN

A QUESTION OF BALANCE:

UNDERSTANDING THE 'ENERGY' OF COMPLEMENTARY THERAPIES

AS WE wind up this exploration of the world of alternative therapies—which can only begin to open up the questions—it is important to take a step back so that we may appreciate the importance of 'energy' in healing. While there is no denying that 'energy' holds an integral and important place in mind, body, spirit medicine, what exactly does the word mean? 'Energy healing' is a phrase that seems to be a catch-all for many people. It is a phrase used equally by those who are good advocates for complementary therapies, those who wish to know more about them, and, unfortunately, by those who have not a clue what they are talking about. The difficulty is that 'energy' conjures up meanings that seem to be limitless—in any context you like. Yet it is a serious concept, and while meanings and applications of the word are diverse in complementary therapies, it is nonetheless important to examine some of them.

Energy is in all of nature; and as we are part of

nature, we are also energetic in our own nature. Different traditions give different slants on this concept; it is a matter of perspective. Thus, in an effort to unravel this picture we'll start right at the top, with energy as 'spirit'.

The concepts of energy and spirit have at many times been interchangeable, not least in the classical and Judaeo-Christian perspectives. In Chapter One, we saw that for Hippocrates, the awareness and well-being of one's spiritual body was as important as the mind and physical body. Hahnemann, in his declaration regarding the cause of illness and disease, brought the Hippocratic philosophy of spirit and healing into the nineteenth century, and Edward Bach carried it forward into the twentieth.

Bach took Hahnemann's philosophy to a deeper level through his writings by constantly reminding us that listening to our divine wisdom is all-important in our healing process. For Bach, intuition is the voice of the soul. He said, 'Disease is the result in the physical body of the resistance of the personality to the guidance of the soul'.* Thus, the spiritual aspect of our wellbeing lies in great part in training ourselves to listen to what our body is telling us through our intuition. However, healing is not only about listening to what our body is trying to tell us through our spiritual intuition, it is also about transition and transformation. James Baltzell, M.D., whose views we heard earlier, says: 'Healing is related to what is going on spiritually, making your body more comfortable as you go through the difficult transits of lessons in this life.' The concept of healing energy has much to do with our relationship to our spirit.

'Spiritual energy' is not exclusive to these perspectives alone. In THE TIBETAN BOOK OF LIVING AND DYING, Sogyal Rinpoche reminds us that to follow the path of our spiritual wisdom has never been more difficult than now; we do not live in a world that supports it. We live in a world that seems to be anchored in the mind, rather than in our spiritual body, and yet operating from our spiritual self is now imperative as never before. As he remarks, 'Spiritual vision is not an elitist luxury, but vital to our survival'. Thus, in complementary medicine, the health of the spiritual self is an important element in our quest for wellbeing in body and mind.

Working to build a solid connection to our spiri-

*Howard and Ramsell, ORIGINAL WRITINGS OF EDWARD BACH. p. 44.

tual self, along with many of the other elements we find in complementary medicine, is itself a process. The good news, however, lies in the variety of ways there are to establish this connection—something for everyone. I mentioned that contemplative prayer and the various approaches to meditation are two of the easiest paths. Classes in yoga often teach meditation as part of the practice, but joining a meditation group is a good way to become familiar and comfortable with the techniques involved. There are many good teachers, and there is no single method of meditation that is 'the one'. Explore and experiment. The important thing is that you are comfortable with the particular tradition; otherwise it is a waste of your time.

However, as I have cautioned throughout this book with regard to the choice of practitioners and therapies, when joining any spiritually-oriented group, check it out first. Spiritual practice is no different from any other practice: there are gifted teachers, those who slip off the path, pseudo-'gurus' who are little more than charlatans, and some who are charlatans from the word 'go'.

ENERGY AND HEALING

Let us look at the relationship between our layers of energy and the various therapies that work with them. In this relationship, the energy of healing is directly applied to both the mind and body aspects of the mind–body–spirit model. However, we can also 'feel' shifts in the energy of our spiritual connections. For many people this comes as an awareness of having a 'direct' connection to the Divine. Whether this be experienced as an external or internal connection depends very much on the spiritual culture of the individual. Regardless of this difference, the energetic balance of these fundamentals is interdependent; if one is out of balance, it will affect the degree of harmony between the others. Furthermore, the relationship between energy and our mind and body is both an internal and an external matter.

Practitioners of holistic therapies visualize our energy in layers, as it flows within us and around us, in perpetual connection. In esoteric traditions, this 'envelope' of vital energy surrounds everything in nature, including the human body, and is known as an aura. To clairvoyants, auras manifest as energetic layers of colours. These layers surrounding the body continuously expand and contract, both in the intensity of their colours and in their boundaries.

As we learned in the chapters that focused on traditional Chinese medicine and ayurveda, *qi*, *prana*, or vital life-force flows along the body's meridians. We can consider this particular energy as being external in its availability. This is why practitioners are able to remove energy blockages along these channels or meridians through therapies such as acupuncture, with the use of needles, and various forms of acupressure, through the hands. Additional therapies that are more 'physical' in nature includes reflexology, which works on pressure points of the feet, and various postures in yoga that can revitalize energy through redirection.

There are also forms of energy therapies that involve minimal physical touch, but nonetheless have been shown as extremely effective. Somewhat similar to older forms of healing such as 'laying-on of hands', they include therapies such as Reiki, Therapeutic Touch and Healing Touch (itself a variant of Therapeutic Touch). Reiki, which is a popular form of bio-energetic healing, boasts over 200,000 practitioners worldwide.*

Regardless of which energy therapy you choose, there is a basic exchange of energetic 'intent' between patient and healer. Thus, the goal of the practitioner is to use his or her energy to remove blockages in the flow of the patient's energy fields. In general, the practitioner uses hand movements along the patient's body in order to 'smooth out' the energetic fields. While it is vital in work such as this that the spiritual, emotional, and physical balance and intent on the part of the practitioner be clear and in balance, this is true of all relationships between practitioner and patient, in complementary medicine. Otherwise, any negativity

*Trivieri and Anderson, p. 132

Chakra	Energetic Center/ Physical Location	Mental/Emotional Issues
First	Base of Spine	Survival
Second	Sexual organs	Creativity, internal view of our individual value
Third	Solar Plexus (gut)	Our value in the external world
Fourth	Heart, Lungs,	Love and compassion, grief
Fifth	Throat	Ability to speak our truth
Sixth	Brow	Intuition
Seventh	Crown (above the head)	Faith, spirituality: 'unconditional knowing'

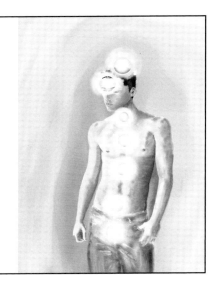

will have an undesired effect upon the patient.

Energetic or massage therapies that focus on our energy fields come under the general category of 'bodywork'. This sub-field of complementary therapies is vast and offers a variety of approaches and methods deserving serious exploration.

No discussion on mind–body–spirit medicine would be complete without at least a brief visit to the subject of chakras. The concept of the chakras is anchored in the ancient yogic tradition within Hinduism and, later, Buddhism. There are extensive authoritative works on the subject of the chakras: what they are, what they do, and how they affect us. As always in subjects of this nature, there are subtle variations in philosophy.

To put it simply, the chakras are seven major centres in the body (along with hundreds of minor ones) that continually vibrate as they function. What they do is to process the various layers of energy within and around us. Their relationship to our physical body is through the pathways of our central nervous system, which lie along our spinal column. Furthermore, each *chakra* represents not only energetic centres but also emotional core issues that are part of the human nature, as outlined in the chart on the previous page.

When we move into distressed emotional states, consciously or unconsciously, negative energy initiates patterns of contraction within the *chakras* and our energetic layers. Like a pebble tossed into a pond of still water, this action reverberates throughout the layers and the disruptive permutations tend to be perpetuated. As we have learned in previous chapters, medical traditions of the East teach that the ultimate result of blockages to positive energetic flow is illness and disease—and so do the spiritual philosophies. Conversely, when we experience positive emotional states, the *chakras* intensify and expand into harmonic balance.

As we are spirit in body, our soul is constantly pushing us toward this harmony between the centres, with the goal of bringing the chakras into full expansion and expression, for our highest good. The process of soul growth is one that leads us, by experience, through the delicate intricacies of emotional balance. Thus, the state of contraction and expansion within the *chakras* provides us yet another map to guide us in our healing process.

KEY POINTS FOR CHAPTER SEVEN:

1. Energy and spirit are often interchangeable in the Judaeo-Christian culture. Access to these is through contemplative prayer or meditation.
2. The practice of meditation is found in many cultures with varying approaches. There is no single 'right' method.
3. Esoteric philosophy teaches that layers of energy, sometimes called 'auras', surround our bodies.
4. These layers require balancing, best accomplished through various types of energetic bodywork.
5. We also possess seven major energetic centres within our body and aura, known as *chakras*. Our emotional states affect their contraction or expansion.
6. Balance of our energy centres externally and internally is the key to overall wellness and manifestation of our highest purpose.

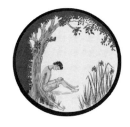

CHAPTER EIGHT

THE NEXT 'RIGHT STEP'

WE HAVE now had a look at the basic philosophy of complementary medicine and some of its major therapies, should you wish to make some changes in how you work with your body, mind and spirit. However, the title of these final pages indicates a departure point for your exploration into the disicplines available. As I mentioned at the start, the intent of this book is to allow you to look out of the usual box and into the wider world of holistic therapies, rather than to provide an in-depth look at the myriad available. Well-known disciplines that space constrictions have not let me examine include therapies such as aromatherapy, sound therapy, colour therapy, crystal healing and magnetic therapy.

Psychotherapy, once the poor relation of Psychiatry, has now evolved beyond 'talk therapy' into various techniques of art therapy, dream therapy, drama therapy and dance therapy. These therapies represent just a very few of the choices available. You will find the addresses listed in 'Selected Resources for Further Study' a helpful place to start if you wish to investigate them.

Regardless of which of the therapies appeal to you, it cannot be emphasized enough that *we are spirit in body*. Preferring intuitive awareness to Cartesian rationalism, all complementary therapies start from this point. We are in body to participate in the process of manifesting our highest purpose; and in order to do this, we must listen with our soul wisdom, our intuition.

Internal harmony with our Divine Self, and the external harmony of universal connection, is an ideal for all humanity. While our soul holds this wisdom, some of us—most of us—have disconnected from it in our frenzy to speed toward and through the wonders of technology. The ancients (and as we have seen, gifted individuals in our own time) intuitively knew that in truth nature is symbiotic with our soul's agenda. They knew that all life-energy is connected. They knew that the divinity of nature enfolds and balances us on all levels. Traditional Chinese medicine and ayurveda gained their healing wisdom by observing the flow and disruptions of nature. Healers such as Hahnemann, Schuessler and Bach knew that nature's resources could assist us in healing mind, body and spirit.

While these elements are very much part of the larger picture, we must not forget that our healing process requires our participation. Furthermore, we should not shun the enormous value of modern medical technology and those who are skilled in practising it. As I stated at the beginning, incorporating complementary medicine into your lifestyle is about inclusion, not exclusion. It is about integration; internally, externally—universally!

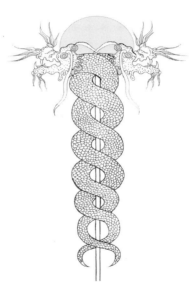

SELECTED FURTHER READING

Bach, Edward. *Collected Writings of Edward Bach,* ed. Julian Barnard. London: Ashgrove Publishing, 1987.

Ballentine, Rudolph. *Radical Healing: Integrating the World's Great Therapeutic Traditions to create a New Transformative Medicine.* New York: Harmony, 1999.

Barnard, Julian. *Bach Flower Remedies: Form & Function,* Hereford: Flower Remedy Programme, 2002.

Beinfield, Harriet, L.Ac., and Korngold, Efrem, L.Ac., O.M.D. *Between Heaven and Earth: A Guide to Chinese Medicine,* New York: Balantine Books, 1992.

Stephen Cummings, M.D., and Dana Ullman, M.P.H. *Everybody's Guide to Homeopathic Medicines.* Los Angeles: Jeremy P. Tarcher, 1991.

Chopra, Deepak, M.D. *Ageless Body, Timeless Mind.* New York: Three Rivers Press, 1998; London: Rider, 2003.

Dossey, Larry M.D. *Healing Beyond the Body,* Boston: Shambala, 2003.

Gerber, Richard. *Vibrational Medicine for the Twenty-First Century: The Complete Guide to Energy Healing and Spiritual Transformation.* New York: Eagle Book-Harper Collins, 2000.

Gordon, James M.D. *Manifesto for a New Medicine.* Reading, Mass.: Perseus Books, 1996.

Hay, Louise. *You Can Heal Your Life.* Santa Monica, Ca.: Hay House, 1984

Howard, Judy, and John Ramsell. *The Original Writings of Edward Bach.* Saffron Walden, Essex: C.W. Daniel Co., Ltd., 1990.

Kaptchuk, Ted J. OMD *The Web That Has No Weaver: Understanding Chinese Medicine.* Chicago: Contemporary Books, 2000.

Kornfield, Jack. *A Path With Heart: A Guide Through the Perils and Promises of Spiritual Life.* New York: Bantam, 1993

Lad, Vasant, M.D. *Ayurveda: The Science of Self-Healing.* Santa Fe, NM: Lotus Press 1984.

Mack, Gaye. *Igniting Soul Fire, Spiritual Dimensions of the Bach Flower Remedies,* London: Polair Publishing, 2004

Morrison, Judith H. *The Book of Ayurveda, A Holistic Approach to Health and Longevity,* New York: Fireside, 1995

Myss, Caroline. *Anatomy of Spirit.* New York: Harmony, 1996.

Rinpoche, Sogyal. *The Tibetan Book of Living and Dying,* ed. Patrick Gaffney and Andrew Harvey. San Francisco: Harper Collins, 1993.

Teasdale, Wayne. *The Mystic Heart.* Novato, Ca.: New World Library, 2001.

Scheffer, Mechthild. *Bach Flower Therapy.* Rochester, Vt.: Inner Traditions, 1987.

Larry Trivieri, Jr. and John W. Anderson, Eds. *Alternative Medicine, The Definitive Guide* Berkeley, Ca.: Celestial Arts. 2002

Weeks, Nora. *The Medical Discoveries of Edward Bach, Physician: What the Flowers do for the Human Body.* Saffron Walden, Essex: C.W. Daniel Co., Ltd., 1973.

SELECTED FURTHER RESOURCES

1. AMERICAN ASSOCIATION OF
   ORIENTAL MEDICINE
   PO Box 162340
   Sacramento, CA 95816
   www.aaom.org

2. AMERICAN COLLEGE OF
   TRADITIONAL CHINESE
   MEDICINE
   455 Arkansas Street
   San Francisco, CA 94107
   www.actcm.org

2. AYURVEDIC INSTITUTE
   11311 Menaul Blvd. N.E.
   Albuquerque, NM. 87112
   www.ayurveda.com

3. NATIONAL CENTER FOR
   HOMEOPATHY(U.S.)
   801 North Fairfax, Suite 306
   Alexandria, Va. 22314
   www.homeopathic.org

4. BRITISH HOMEOPATHY AND
   COMPLEMENTARY MEDICINE

520 Washington Blvd., Suite 423
Marina Del Rey, Ca. 90202
and
Endeavour House
80 High Street
Egham, Surrey, Tw20 9he
England
www.britinsthom.com

5. DR EDWARD BACH CENTRE
   Mount Vernon, Bakers Lane,
   Sotwell, Oxon, OX10 0PZ, UK
   England
   www.bachcentre.com

6. HEALING HERBS LTD.
   Healing Herbs Ltd
   PO Box 65
   Hereford, HR2 0DX
   England
   www.healing-herbs.co.uk

7. FLOWER ESSENCE SOCIETY
   P.O. Box 459
   Nevada City, Ca. 95959
   www.flowersociety.org

8. PERELANDRA, LTD.
   P.O. Box 3603
   Warrenton, Va. 20188
   www. Perelandra-ltd.com

9. NATURESBRIDGE, Inc.
   471 Old Barn Road
   Barrington, Il. 60010
   www.naturesbridge.com

10. POLAIR PUBLISHING
    P. O. Box 34886
    London W8 6YR
    www.polairpublishing.co.uk

11. OTHER USEFUL LINKS
    Traditional Chinese Medicine:
    www.rchm.co.uk
    www.jcm.co.uk
    Ayurveda
    www.bbc.co.uk/health/healthy_living/
    complementary_medicine/tradi-
    tional_ayurvedic.shtml
    Other therapies
    www.crystalandhealing.com